fitness

for

BOOMERS

Disclaimer:
The intention of this publication is solely informational and educational.
Consult your physician or primary health provider, before beginning any
exercise program. The author and publisher disclaim any liability, personal
or professional, resulting from the use / application or misapplication of
any of the information in this publication.

STOP!

**If you develop chest pains, dizziness or other dangerous condition while
doing any of the exercises or activities stop and contact your physician**

Order this book online at www.trafford.com
or email orders@trafford.com

Most Trafford titles are also available at major online book retailers.

Printed in the United States of America.

ISBN: 978-1-4120-5380-8 (sc)

Trafford rev. 03/16/2011

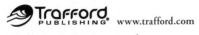 www.trafford.com

North America & international
toll-free: 1 888 232 4444 (USA & Canada)
phone: 250 383 6864 ♦ fax: 812 355 4082

Acknowledgements

Thank you to my wife Patty. Through the 25+ years we have been married she has been my rock and my anchor; especially through the 7+ years it has taken me to complete this project. The photos of Patty and me in this book will show you a few of the incredible places we have traveled together always getting involved in great adventures. Our house looks like a museum of travels with artifacts from Europe, Asia, all over America, South America and the Arctic...what an adventure!

Thank you to my father Gerard Cook. His example of completing a book when he was 88 years old was an example of focus and hard work for me to follow.

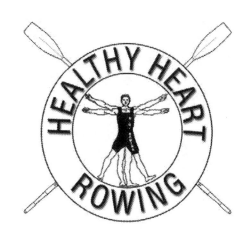

Thank you to my daughter Petra Elke (Cook) Townsend MD who is pictured often in this tome rowing with me at various events. Come back and row with me sometime.

Thank you to Mary Aveni who has been extremely patient with my starts and stops during our 7 year friendship working on this book...she never gave up...amazing!!!

Thank you to Kristina (Chambers) Hill whose original art work was much of the inspiration for this book.

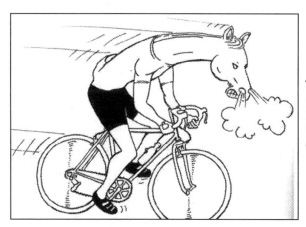

Thank you to Robert Rivollier; Medical Director, Mont Faucon Hospital, France, for his art work and inspiration.

SPECIAL THANK YOU TO CONCEPT 2 ROWING

A very special THANK YOU!!! to Concept 2 Rowing. The Concept 2 Rowing folks have helped me to maintain my sanity through use of their rowing machine over a period of 25 + years.

During my military time I used the C-2 "ERG" to train on while reducing my blood pressure and stress rate!

I used the ERG to keep me in shape through Desert Storm deployments to South Com, Hurricane duty here in Florida, making preparations to deploy the RED HORSE unit to Iraq and Afghanistan and a host of other highly stressfull periods.

Since I have retired Concept 2 has anointed me as a C-2 Master Rowing Instructor and has sent me around the country to teach individuals to become Indoor Rowing Instructors.

Then: when I told the C-2 folks I wanted to use their data to write a book they said YES! It is Amazing.

I cannot say enough good about Concept 2.

Use their products, buy their ERG, become healthy and fit rowing as often as possible...maybe even EVERY DAY!!!

Contents

"How old would you be if you did not know when you were born"

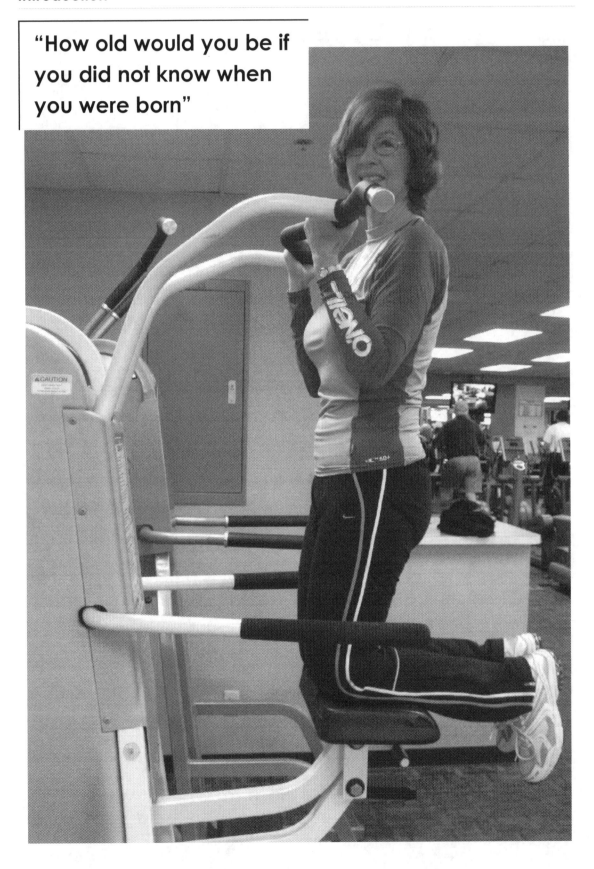

Introduction

One of the healthiest things you can do for yourself is EXERCISE!

Regular scheduled exercise and physical activity are very important to the health and independence of individuals as they grow older. The American College of Sports Medicine recently published data showing that NOT exercising is a risky behavior!

Our goal is to help people look better, feel better and achieve a healthier lifestyle!

The reason Patty and I decided to write this book is to provide an easily used system of exercises that we have used for many years to keep ourselves healthy.

Usually, when people age and lose their ability to do things on their own, it does not happen just because they have increased in age in days, months and years. More likely, they have allowed themselves to become INACTIVE. Older, inactive adults lose ground in four areas that are important for staying healthy and independent: aerobic endurance, strength, balance and flexibility.

These four activities:
Aerobic Endurance; Strength; Balance and Flexibility... are AGE DEFYING ACTIVITIES!

The Surgeon General of the United States said:

"The good news...is that people can benefit from even moderate levels of physical activity."

Introduction

Do not despair, scientific research suggests that you can maintain and even partly restore endurance, strength, balance and flexibility by exercising. Additional improvements can be made through everyday physical activities such as walking and gardening and through many other everyday activities as well as the activities Patty and I include... Bicycling and Rowing.

What may seem like very small changes in exercise and physical activity...can make a BIG IMPACT!!

Getting Into Action

The exercises Patty and I have chosen here use equipment available in most YMCA and other public type gyms. Indoor Rowers made by Concept 2 Rowing ® and bicycles (stationary or non-stationary) are available for use just about anywhere. We have used rubber-band type resistance equipment for strength training.

However, you may continue to be afraid that physical activity could harm you. You could also feel you must join a gym or purchase expensive equipment...not true. You could also feel embarrassed because you feel people must look good in exercise clothes! You can bicycle on just about any bicycle anywhere in the world. Indoor rowers can be found through, www.concept2.com web site to locate Indoor Rowers in your area.

Success comes by increasing your physical activity by exercising and by using your own muscle power!

Who Can Exercise?

Recent studies by The American College of Sports Medicine www.acsm-healthfitness.org indicate that older adults hurt their health far more by NOT EXERCISING than by exercising!!!

Therefore, Patty and I recommend that older Americans stay as physically active as they possibly can.

Lack of exercise and poor diet are the second leading cause of death in the USA. Smoking is #1 cause!

WORDS IN THIS BOOK

Here are some of the more important words used in our book explained as they will be used:

Aerobics – or aerobic exercises. These are terms coined by Dr. Cooper in his 1968 landmark book "AEROBICS". We will refer to these exercises as "endurance training activities". These activities increase your heart rate and breathing for an extended period of time.
See the section on ENDURANCE TRAINING: Bicycling and Rowing.

Cardiovascular refers to the human heart and the body circulatory system.

Frailty has many meanings…In our book we use it to mean a physical condition caused by severe muscle loss as seen in individuals who have been inactive for many years. Frail people have great loss of strength and may not be able to perform everyday tasks.

Resistance Training…In our book we use resistance training when we speak about training that might otherwise be referred to as "weight lifting" training. Patty and I have used "Rubber Band" resistance training for many years to build muscles and maintain muscle strength and balance.

Physical activity / Exercise…Exercise is physical activity that is planned.

What Can Exercise Do For Me?

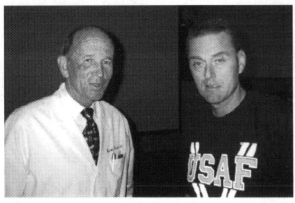

Doctor Ken Cooper and Colonel Jere Cook, US Air Force (retired)

Both the term Aerobics and the specific exercise method were developed by Kenneth H. Cooper M.D., an exercise physiologist, and Col. Pauline Potts, a physical therapist, both in the United States Air Force.

In an amazing stroke of "fate", I stopped in San Antonio, Texas in September 1970 while on my way to Air Force Flight School in Del Rio, Texas. In San Antonio, I purchased a copy of Dr. Cooper's 1968 book "AEROBICS"!

Dr. Cooper, an avowed exercise enthusiast, was personally and professionally puzzled about why some people with excellent muscular strength were still prone to poor performance at tasks such as long-distance running, swimming, and bicycling. He began measuring systematic human performance using a bicycle ergometer, and began measuring sustained performance in terms of a person's ability to use oxygen. When I attended his Cooper Institute for Aerobics Research (CIAR) I used the same type of bicycle ergometer. His groundbreaking book, *AEROBICS*, was published in 1968, and included scientific exercise programs using running, walking, swimming and bicycling. The book came at a fortuitous historical moment, when increasing weakness and inactivity in the general population was causing a perceived need for increased exercise. It became a bestseller. Cooper's data provided the scientific baseline for almost all modern aerobics programs, most of which are based on oxygen-consumption equivalency.

The training Patty and I suggest in this book is based on the same oxygen-consumption equivalency for endurance training. However, we recommend the use of the Concept2 Ergometer (C2-ERG) as the training machine. We recommend the C2-ERG because we feel we achieve a better whole body muscle exercise at the same time we achieve significant Endurance (cardio-vascular) training.

What Can Endurance, Strength, Balance and Stretching Exercises Do For Me?

By this time in the 21st Century most people have a good idea EXERCISE is probably good for them. However, in an article in ACSM's (American College of Sports Medicine) Health and Fitness Journal, Sept/Oct 2009, somehow, many older adults have been omitted from this picture...until only recently. www.acsm-healthfitness.org

In 2010 a new picture is growing out of research that older people with many different physical conditions have many positive benefits to gain from staying physically active. As we have read already...they have much to lose if they become physically inactive.

No Age Limit To Benefits from Exercise

During my studies to complete my Master's Degree, I discovered new data from studies in Italy and France that individuals in their 80's and 90's could increase their strength and physical stamina through routine daily exercise. Some in their 90's could regain the ability to walk without assistance!

So, exercise is not just for old folks in the younger age ranges who live independently and can go on brisk jogs. Staying physically active along with regular exercise can prevent or delay many diseases and disabilities as people grow older. For people who already present diseases and disabilities there is usually improvement in health if the exercise is done on a routine schedule and is maintained over a long period of time.

Activities That Improve Ability and Health

There are four Age Defying activities that help older adults gain health benefits.
AGE DEFYING Endurance training will increase your breathing and heart rate...your cardiovascular system. Endurance exercises strengthen and improve the health of your heart, lungs and circulatory system. With increased endurance you will increase your feeling of health, keep yourself healthier and improve your stamina for activities of daily living (ADL's) that will allow you to live and accomplish things on your own... ADL's include, shopping, climbing stairs and going to the grocery store. Endurance training may also delay or even prevent many aging related diseases. The most common diseases of aging are diabetes, colon cancer, stroke and heart disease. It has been scientifically shown

that endurance exercise can increase healthful aging and reduce hospitalization rates.

AGE DEFYING Strength Training will build muscles and so much more than just make you stronger. Increasing muscle mass throughout your body will give you more strength to accomplish ADL's each day on your own. Studies have shown that even small increases in muscle mass can make big differences in daily living especially for frail individuals. The very act of increasing your muscle mass will increase your metabolism and that will assist weight control. As we all age, anything we can do to keep a reasonable weight will assist to keep our blood sugar in balance and reduce risk of diabetes. As Patty and I look around at some of our aging contemporaries, we see creeping obesity setting in and the on-set of Type-2 diabetes. In most cases, the diabetes is caused by sedentary life style coupled with a diet high in sugars and saturated fats.
Another big plus...strength training has been shown to slow, prevent and possibly even reverse the effects of osteoporosis. Among the many women and men I train in my Masters Rowing courses, one of the biggest concerns for those over 60 is prevention of osteoporosis.
The definition of osteoporosis is literally "porous bone" a disease that makes bones easy to break. Unfortunately, genetics is a major factor in the chemistry that determines the degree of bone deterioration...we are born with tendencies that cannot be changed. However, scientific research now has shown us that people who are active in childhood and continue to stay active through adulthood have thicker bones! Now in the past 10 years we have proven that exercise does make a difference throughout life. www.healthylivingbooks.com   Exercise for Osteoporosis; Daniels, MA.

AGE DEFYING Balance Training helps prevent a common problem among older people...falling! Loss of independence in older age is caused most by falling often due to simple balance challenges. Broken hips and broken bones are the major result of even the simplest fall. Balance exercises, along with general strength exercises build up muscles in the legs. Even the simplest balance exercise of briefly balancing on one leg will assist muscles to balance the body.

AGE DEFYING Flexibility Exercises help the body remain limber by stretching the muscles and tissues that hold the body's bone structure together. A general course of stretching as described in the book, along with stretches prescribed by physical therapist help prevent injuries from occurring. When injuries do occur: stretches will often be prescribed by physical therapists to aid in recovery. Patty and I use stretching to help us stay limber and less "fall susceptible".

In my Master's Degree training and at The Cooper Institute (CIAR) we studied 90 year old physically frail individuals, all frail from inactivity, _who more than doubled their strength through simple exercises in a short amount of time._ This allowed them to rise from a chair without assistance from another person!

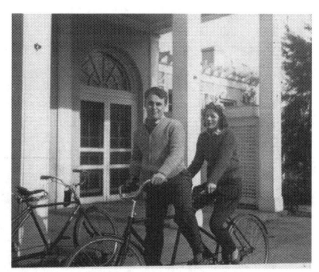

60 YEARS + Exercising…It's the way to GO!

Several years ago I asked my father to write a few lines about how he was coping with my mother's death and his seemingly failing health and strength along with reduced ADLs. What I received was a fantastic statement on life, helping a failing spouse AND recovering his strength and health at age 85! Here is part of "Gerard's Story".

Dear (Colonel) Jere: I have enclosed this photo of your mother and I to encourage you and Patty to continue riding YOUR tandem. This photo was shot in Washington D. C. in February 1942.

So what is happening to me as I enter my 85th year?   The legs are giving out! Walking becomes difficult. Falling unexpectedly usually happened without warning. Constant imbalance rules as soon as I leave a sitting or sleeping position.

Now that I have slipped into this dangerous way of life, I am aghast! How could I do this so easily!? And, not realize months ago this pitiful slide into almost helplessness might become permanent! Not only permanent…but could lead to an early death!

It takes months (in my case several years) to realize the gradual loss of self control. In today's world it can indeed become not only frightening, but saddening. What happens to me now? It seemed no problem to me to take proper care of my wife, for ten years as she slipped through various stages of dementia.

Introduction

Our life together came to an end when Virginia passed away. A stunning blow. The grief is unrelenting. The constant care I had conducted was gone!

My awareness of increasing frailness was pushed into the back of my brain. MD friends, family observers and friends offered comments such as mostly "old age" creeping up! But I asked myself...was it? Maybe. Maybe not. It dawned on me to take a better look. An assessment for ADL's quickly showed I needed improvement.

I had been lucky to have been on the board of the Institute of Physical Medicine and Rehabilitation (IPMR) for 48 years. I approached the IPMR Staff and began a program of exercise four days a week for Endurance, Strength, Balance and Flexibility training. How long will I be doing this? I use the Tread Mill (endurance) Stationary Bicycle (endurance) Chest Press and Leg Press Machines (Strength) Modified Wobble Board (Balance) and Yoga Stretches (Flexibility) with the Instructor. So HOW LONG will I be doing this training. Hopefully for another 20 years...until I am at least 105!

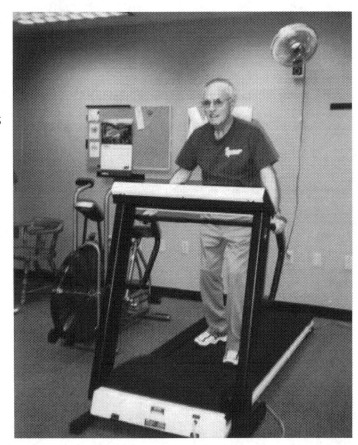

Dad!

Sun Salutation

"It is hard to get much done one little step at a time. However, it is impossible to accomplish anything significant without going one little step at a time."
   Confucius

The Sun Salutation is a series of Yoga poses that have been used for centuries. The poses are flowing poses that are often performed as a morning wake-up routine or in preparation for bicycling, kayaking, rowing or any other activity. The poses flow quickly or slowly from one pose to the next. Done quickly repeatedly the Sun Salutation appears to be a dance.

As my physical therapist at Mayo Clinic told me…"We see people in here every day who have blown out their backs bending over to pick up the morning newspaper in their driveways because they did not warm up their body even marginally before trekking out for the newspaper!" Reread this again and remember to warm up by getting blood flowing to your back and extremities before getting that morning paper.

This series of Yoga poses enhances flexibility of the spine, legs and chest while strengthening the arms, shoulders and enhancing your body's sense of balance and coordination. (The number one fear of most people over age 60 is falling…balance training in this and other Yoga poses can mitigate the fear of falling.)

Patty and I recommend you try to hold each pose for 5 to 15 seconds when first learning the sequence. Ultimately, we want you to be able to hold this stretch / yoga pose for at least 30 seconds. There are 12 poses in the famous Yoga poses sequence. Once you have mastered these poses you can move through them quickly perhaps as fast as finishing in 2 or 3 minutes.

In this series of Yoga poses as well as all the exercises herein REMEMBER TO BREATHE when performing any exercise or stretch! This may seem strange, however, many exercisers forget to breathe when performing stretches, endurance work and strength training.

PRAYER POSE

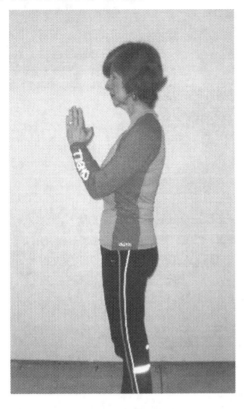

1. Stand tall with feet at hip width.

2. Gently press palms together in prayer position.

3. Inhale deeply.

MOUNTAIN POSE

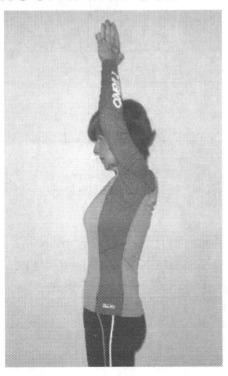

1. Exhale as you reach upwards with both arms.

FORWARD POSE

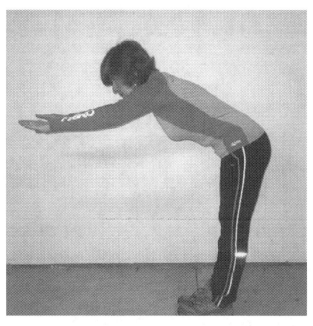

1. Inhale as you bend your body forward.

2. Lower your torso, with your arms reaching forward.

3. Bring your hands to the floor as the back bends slightly.

LUNGE POSITION

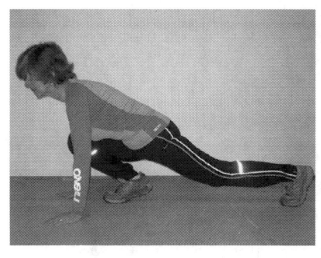

1. Bend both knees as your hands reach the floor and support your body.

2. Exhale as you step back with your right foot until the left knee is as close to a right angle as possible. REMEMBER to breathe!

3. Allow your mid-section to rest against the top of your left thigh.

PLANK POSITION

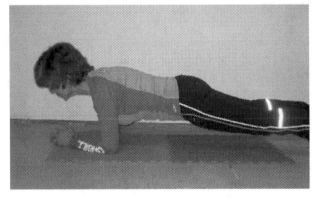

1. Move gently from your hands holding your body off the floor to resting on your elbows.

2. Inhale as you rest on your elbows to support your body's weight.

3. Move gently from your elbows holding the body off the floor back to straight arms holding your body off floor.

GRASSHOPPER POSITION

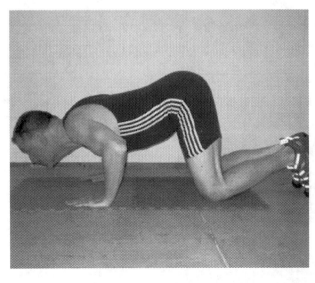

1. From the straight arm Plank position, bend at the elbow and knees.

2. Exhale as you allow your body to lower towards the floor as close as is comfortable for you to lower yourself.

UPWARD FACING DOG

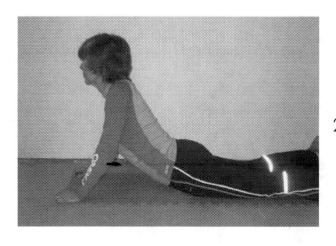

1. Inhale as you press upward and forward as your legs and arms straighten from the Grasshopper Position.

2. Keep the thigh muscles contracted to help support your body.

DOWNWARD FACING DOG

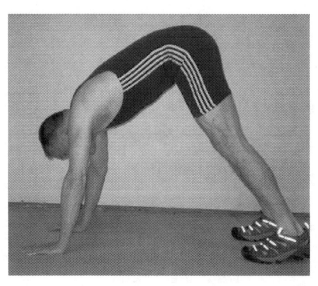

1. Exhale as you push your body backward on to your hands and feet as the legs, arms and back straighten.

2. Push your heels to the floor while maintaining straight legs and push your hips away from your hands.

3. Point the buttocks toward the ceiling.

RETURN TO LUNGE POSITION

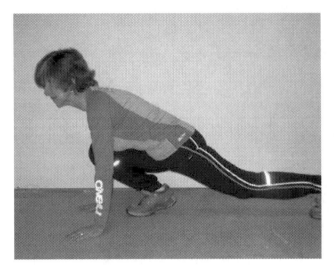

1. Return to lunge position with opposite leg forward hands flat on floor.

2. Step forward and inhale as you move into lunge with right foot until right knee is set.

3. Allow your midsection to rest against right knee.

DEEP FORWARD BEND

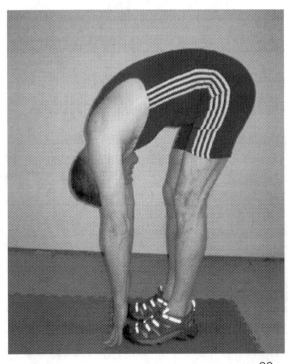

1. Bring rear foot forward from lunge position to have both legs parallel.

2. Exhale as you bend your body forward

3. Inhale as torso is raised, keep arms parallel with the spine.

20

MOUNTAIN POSE: begin return to start

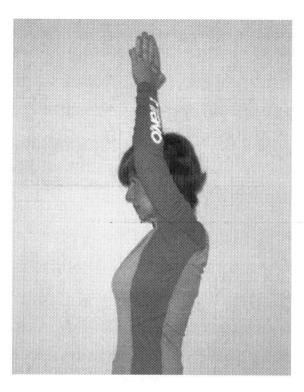

1. Exhale as you reach upwards with both arms.

2. Hold for 5 breaths at top of pose, then continue with next pose.

PRAYER POSE: restart sequence

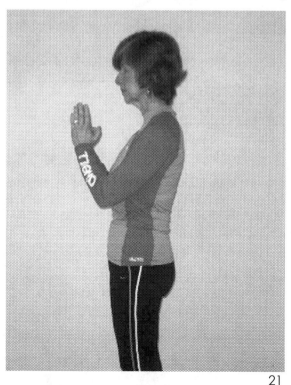

1. Stand tall with feet at hip width.

2. Gently press palms together in prayer position.

3. Inhale deeply.

4. Repeat entire sequence with gentle flowing movements.

Rowing

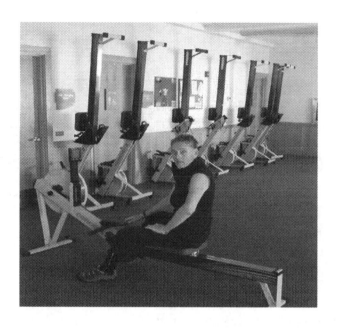

Indoors and on the Water

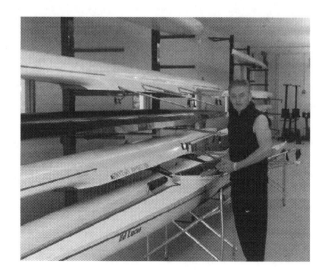

WHY Patty and I RECOMMEND YOU ROW FOR HEALTH AT ANY AGE!

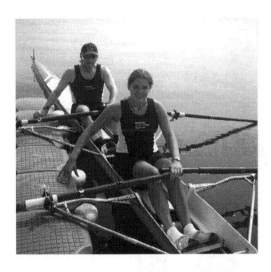

Author Jere Cook(Colonel (ret) and daughter Doctor Petra (Cook) Townsend, M. D. ready to launch to the race course at New Smyrna Beach, Florida circa 1995.

1. Rowing exercises all of your major muscle groups: legs, arms, back, buttocks and abdomen.

2. Rowing moves your body through a very wide range of motion. When you row on the water or on the Concept 2 Indoor Rower, your muscles and joints move and stretch safely through a greater range of motion than most other exercises. This greater range of motion helps promote flexibility and mobility...very important issues to me at age 62!

3. Rowing is an aerobic exercise, and can be an anaerobic exercise as well as strength conditioning.

4. Rowing is an incredible calorie burner. Check on the Concept 2 web site to see how rowing compares with bicycling.

5. Rowing is impact free...a very important point for people my age.

6. Rowing is very time efficient. You do not require a large amount of time.

7. You can row inside, outside on the Concept 2 rower or in a real rowing shell!

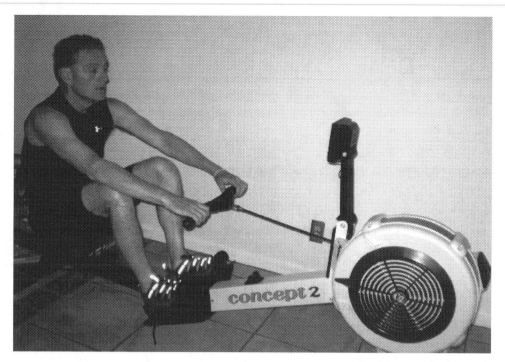

From my own individual history of being in a VERY stressful position as the Commanding Colonel of a Combat Engineer Squadron, rowing provided me with very real benefits:

1. Reduced stress and anxiety.

2. Kept me in shape for Combat training and deployments.

3. Weight control and blood pressure reduction.

4. Provided exercise that was injury free.

5. Exercise to help me clear my mind and concentrate on something fun.

HOW TO START ROWING ON THE INDOOR ROWER

As a Concept 2 Master Indoor Rowing Trainer and a U. S. Rowing Association Level 3 Coach, I teach a large number of people how to row on the Indoor Rower and on the water. For the purposes of this book I will discuss rowing on the Concept 2 Indoor Rower only.

Concept 2 trainers recommend that if you have questions about the correct technique that you call Concept 2 toll free at 800-245-5676 and request a free technique poster or video. We also recommend you have a friend video tape you rowing on the Indoor Rower and compare the video with the poster or video from Concept 2.

If you are lucky enough, you can look on the Concept2 web site for a Concept 2 certified Indoor Rowing Instructor who may be located in your area. Contact this person and have them help you even if it is for only one session.

Very Important Things to Know When You Are Starting

I have many stories, some very humorous, about the mysterious setting of the Damper. The damper is set using the lever on the side of the big wheel. See the Indoor Rower photo diagram elsewhere in the book to locate the damper lever and read about the settings.

When you first start rowing set the damper to between 1 and 3. When you pull on the handle there may not be much resistance…that is ok…the light resistance is where you want to be. Compare it to starting running and buying your 1st pair of running shoes, going out and running 10 miles the first day! **Start slowly…build up slowly…trust me on this one**. Once you get accustomed to the rower and the motion the wheel will spin faster and the resistance will rise.

Start keeping a training log. Concept 2 has Log Books, an electronic logbook system on their web site or you can use a calendar, your own log system, an "APP" or any other means to track your progress and meters. Keep a record and work towards attaining One Million meters…then additional millions!

Another motivational help is to row with a partner and log your meters. It will make your workouts more fun.

Stretch before and after you do your rowing workout

Look for the Stretching on or off the Indoor Rower elsewhere in this book. Warm up for 5 minutes with easy rowing or climbing stairs. Just exercise enough to warm up your body and your muscles.

MODEL D INDOOR ROWER

The Model D delivers proven performance and fitness benefits.

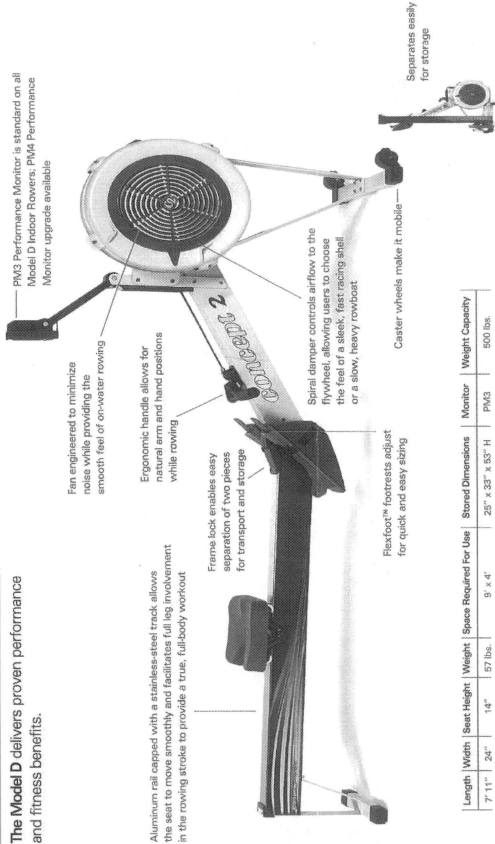

Separates easily for storage

PM3 Performance Monitor is standard on all Model D Indoor Rowers; PM4 Performance Monitor upgrade available

Fan engineered to minimize noise while providing the smooth feel of on-water rowing

Ergonomic handle allows for natural arm and hand positions while rowing

Spiral damper controls airflow to the flywheel, allowing users to choose the feel of a sleek, fast racing shell or a slow, heavy rowboat

Caster wheels make it mobile

Frame lock enables easy separation of two pieces for transport and storage

Flexfoot™ footrests adjust for quick and easy sizing

Aluminum rail capped with a stainless-steel track allows the seat to move smoothly and facilitates full leg involvement in the rowing stroke to provide a true, full-body workout

Length	Width	Seat Height	Weight	Space Required For Use	Stored Dimensions	Monitor	Weight Capacity
7' 11"	24"	14"	57 lbs.	9' x 4'	25" x 33" x 53" H	PM3	500 lbs.

28

How Much Power Should I Put Into My Rowing...PM-2 / 3 Will Tell You

How Much Power Should I Put Into My Piece...PM-2 / 3 Will Tell You

This is a photo of an "Old PM-2" monitor. Even though it is an old model unit it still will explain the concept of how to read what you are doing on the ERG.

-This window tells me I have rowed for 24 seconds...shows total time rowed.

-This window says I am rowing 45 strokes a minute...do not try this! It is too fast for a beginner.

-This window tells me I am rowing 500 meters every one minute and forty two seconds...that is *fast...*

This window shows my heart rate from an optional heart rate monitor.

This window tells me I have rowed 118 meters...if I keep rowing the 1minute and 42 second pace...I will row 500 meters when the time window reads 1min and 42 seconds.

HOW MUCH POWER AND SPEED SHOULD I USE WHEN JUST STARTING?

The rower will row a faster time by pushing harder with the legs.

When you first start rowing learn the technique using the TECHNIQUE REVIEW shown in the rowing section.
We recommend you use the "big window" (500 meter pace) and the SPM (Strokes Per Minute) window as your control system.

Keep your 500 meter pace around 3:00 to 2:30 for the first week of rowing. If you feel comfortable at this pace, then stay at 3:00 to 2:30 until you feel like you can row a faster pace. Your heart rate will quickly tell you how fast you can go.

Regarding the SPM window, many starting rowers are misguided in believing rowing a faster SPM will make them have a faster time and a more productive workout. A wiser rower will know that a faster SPM will tire the rower more quickly and possibly injure the rower. A good SPM starting out is around 20 to 25 SPM.

Technique Review

There are two parts to the rowing stroke, the drive and the recovery, but the movements are blended together to make the stroke smooth and continuous. There should be no stopping at any point in the stroke. Aim for a stroke rate of between 24 and 30 strokes per minute as displayed on the Performance Monitor. Grip should be loose and comfortable; wrists should be level. We suggest that you have someone watch you row and compare your body positions to that shown in the illustrations. Improper technique can result in injury.

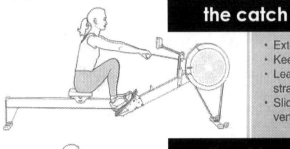

the catch

- Extend your arms straight toward the flywheel.
- Keep your wrists flat.
- Lean your upper body slightly forward with back straight but not stiff.
- Slide forward on the seat until your shins are vertical. (It's OK if heel lifts slightly.)

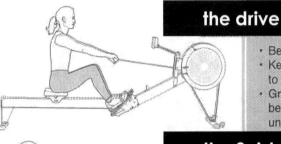

the drive

- Begin the drive by pressing down your legs.
- Keep your arms straight and hold your back firm to transfer your leg power up to the handle.
- Gradually swing back with your upper body, bending your arms amd prying against the legs until you reach a slight backward lean at the finish.

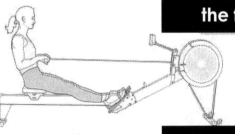

the finish

- Pull handle all the way into your abdomen.
- Straighten your legs.
- Lean your upper body back slightly.

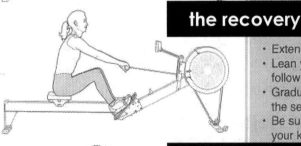

the recovery

- Extend your arms toward the flywheel.
- Lean your upper body forward at the hips to follow the arms.
- Gradually bend your legs to slide forward on the seat.
- Be sure your arms are extended before you bend your knees.

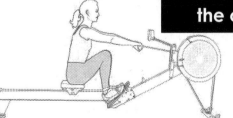

the catch

- Draw your body forward until the shins are vertical.
- Upper body should be leaning forward at the hips.
- Arms should be fully extended.
- You are ready to take the next stroke.

Common Problems to Avoid:
Note that the shadowed figure is in the **incorrect** position.

Technique Review

Common Problem 1: Too Much Forward Reach

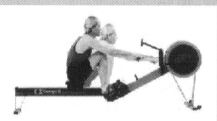

WRONG: The seat nearly hits the heels, the shins are past the vertical, the body leans too far forward, and the head and shoulders drop toward the toes. This puts the body in a weak position for the start of the next stroke.

RIGHT: The seat remains at least 7-10 inches from the heels, the shins are nearly vertical, the body leans comfortably forward, and do not drop the head and shoulders.

Common Problem 2: Rocking On (Opening Back too Early)

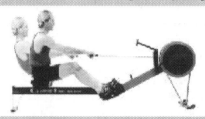

WRONG: The rower pulls the handle by leaning back rather than by pressing the legs. This wastes the power of the legs and may strain the back.

RIGHT: The legs should start the drive with the body still leaning forward. The back then gradually opens, prying against the extended legs.

Common Problem 3: Shooting the Tail (Opening Back Too Late)

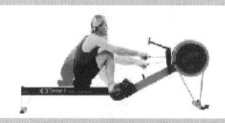

WRONG: The rower starts the drive by extending the legs without moving the handle. The power of the legs is wasted.

RIGHT: The body needs to come along with the legs, thereby transferring the legs' power into the handle. The back then gradually opens, prying against the extended legs. Hips and handle move together.

Common Problem 4: Early Knee Bend on the Recovery

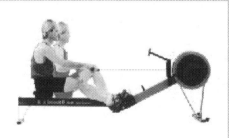

WRONG: On the recovery, the rower lets the knees come up before the arms are fully extended. As a result, either the knees and hands collide (thud!) or the hands are forced to travel upward in a big arc to avoid the knees (unnecessary work for arms!)

RIGHT: The rower should extend the arms completely and lean the upper body forward from the hips BEFORE bending the knees to slide forward. This gets the hands out nicely ahead of the knees.

CONCEPT II INDOOR ROWER PACE CHART

Use this chart to predict your final time or distance for the workouts shown.

Avg pace per 500 m	1000m	2000m	2500m	10,000m	20 min	30 min	60 min
1:28	2:56	5:52	7:20	29:20	6,820	10,230	20,460
1:30	3:00	6:00	7:30	30:00	6,670	10,000	20,000
1:32	3:04	6:08	7:40	30:40	6,520	9,780	19,560
1:34	3:08	6:16	7:50	31:20	6,380	9,570	19,140
1:36	3:12	6:24	8:00	32:00	6,250	9,380	18,760
1:38	3:16	6:32	8:10	32:40	6,120	9,180	18,360
1:40	3:20	6:40	8:20	33:20	6,000	9,000	18,000
1:42	3:24	6:48	8:30	34:00	5,880	8,820	17,640
1:44	3:28	6:56	8:40	34:40	5,770	8,650	17,300
1:46	3:32	7:04	8:50	35:20	5,660	8,490	16,980
1:48	3:36	7:12	9:00	36:00	5,560	8,330	16,660
1:50	3:40	7:20	9:10	36:40	5,450	8,180	16,360
1:52	3:44	7:28	9:20	37:20	5,360	8,040	16,080
1:54	3:48	7:36	9:30	38:00	5,260	7,890	15,780
1:56	3:52	7:44	9:40	38:40	5,170	7,760	15,520
1:58	3:56	7:52	9:50	39:20	5,080	7,630	15,260
2:00	4:00	8:00	10:00	40:00	5,000	7,500	15,000
2:02	4:04	8:08	10:10	40:40	4,920	7,380	14,760
2:04	4:08	8:16	10:20	41:20	4,840	7,260	14,520
2:06	4:12	8:24	10:30	42:00	4,760	7,140	14,280
2:08	4:16	8:32	10:40	42:40	4,690	7,030	14,060
2:10	4:20	8:40	10:50	43:20	4,620	6,920	13,840
2:12	4:24	8:48	11:00	44:00	4,550	6,820	13,640
2:14	4:28	8:56	11:10	44:40	4,480	6,720	13,440
2:16	4:32	9:04	11:20	45:20	4,410	6,620	13,240
2:18	4:36	9:12	11:30	46:00	4,350	6,520	13,040
2:20	4:40	9:20	11:40	46:40	4,290	6,430	12,860
2:22	4:44	9:28	11:50	47:20	4,230	6,340	12,680
2:24	4:48	9:36	12:00	48:00	4,170	6,250	12,500
2:26	4:52	9:44	12:10	48:40	4,110	6,160	12,320
2:28	4:56	9:52	12:20	49:20	4,050	6,080	12,160
2:30	5:00	10:00	12:30	50:00	4,000	6,000	12,000

Use this chart to manage your heart rate using:
Measured Heart Rate per Minute (hr/m) and/or Rate of Preceived Exertion (RPE)

	%hr/m	EXERCISE ZONES										
AGE		30	40	45	50	55	60	65	70	75	80	85
HEART	100%	190	180	175	170	165	160	155	150	145	140	135
		VO 2 MAX (Maximum Effort)										
B	95%	180	171	166	161	157	152	147	142	134	133	128
E								RPE 18 to 20				
A												
T	90%	171	162	158	153	148	144	140	135	130	126	121
S		Anaerobic (Hard Core Training at very high intensity)						RPE 17 to 14				
P	80%	152	144	140	136	132	128	124	120	116	112	108
E		Aerobic (Cardio training / endurance training)						RPE 13 to 11				
R												
M	70%	133	126	123	119	116	112	109	105	101	98	95
I		Weight Control (General Fitness / Fat burn)						RPE 10 to 6				
N	60%	114	108	105	102	99	96	93	90	87	84	81
U												
T	50%	Warm-up and General Maintenance						RPE 6 to 0				
E												

jc2009

How do I use my Heart Rate to manage my workouts?

There are two methods most often used to calculate / measure the amount of exertion you are placing on your body and ultimately your heart. The two methods presented here are named **RPE (Rate of Preceived Exertion) and hr/m Heart Rate Maximum).**

The RPE measurement requires no measurement except your own awareness. The level of effort you feel you are putting into an activity is likely to be the same as a calculated scientific measurement. An example is simple... if your body feels like the exercise you are doing puts a moderate strain on you, measurements of how hard your heart is working would show that your heart is working at a moderate level. This scale is called the BORG Category Rating Scale of **RPE** Rate of Preceived Exertion. The numbers run from 6 to 20. Over many years of experimenting with individuals, the numbers have been correlated to measured **heart rate** they are exercising.

The Heart Rate per Minute **hr/m** method uses measurement of your heart rate taken from your body by measuring your own pulse at your wrist or by using an electronic **heart rate monitor** that records your heart beats and displays the number on a device usually on a watch on your wrist; the electric signal comes from a strap around your chest.

Jere is 62 years old. His upper hr/m number is 148 bpm / his RPE upper numbers are 14 - 17 RPE.

SETTING UP A TRAINING PROGRAM

Determine your Goals

They may be one or more of the following:

- To lose some weight.
- To maintain general health and fitness.
- To aid in rehabilitation.
- To cross-train for another sport.
- To train for competitive rowing.

Choose a Training Program to Meet Your Goals

Here are some basic guidelines for setting up a training program to achieve your goals.

A. WEIGHT LOSS - 60 - 75% Heart Rate Maximum

If weight loss is your goal, then consistency and duration of your workouts will be very important.

Consistency: If possible, set up a regular time to row so that you won't have to make a daily decision about whether and when to row. This will help prevent excuses from interfering with your program. The support of friends and family can be very helpful, too.

Duration: The longer you row at any given intensity level, the more calories you will burn. Rowing at a higher intensity level will also burn calories faster, but you don't want to row so intensely that you can only last for five minutes. Therefore, the best guideline for weight loss is to aim for rows that are at least 30 minutes long, at a "comfortably intense" pace.

Connection to diet: Weight loss should result when your caloric output (exercise) increases while your caloric input (food) decreases or stays the same.

RECOMMENDED WORKOUT FREQUENCY: 5-6 times per week

DURATION: 30-50 minutes

WORK TYPE & INTENSITY: Moderate steady work, able to carry on a conversation; add interval workouts for variety.

SAMPLE WORKOUTS:

- 5,000-7000 meter row
- 10,000 meter row
- 30 minute row
- 1 minute harder, 1 minute easier for at least 20 minutes total
- 2-3 moderate 10-minute pieces with 2 minutes easy in between
- a 30-40 minute piece with 20-30 hard strokes every 5 minutes

B. GENERAL HEALTH AND FITNESS

The guidelines for general health and fitness are that one should exercise at least three times per week for 30 minutes.

FREQUENCY: 3-5 times per week; alternate with other types of exercise if desired.

DURATION: At least 20 minutes total.

WORKTYPE & INTENSITY: Moderate steady work, moderate interval workouts for variety. Use a target heart rate if you have a heart rate monitor.

SAMPLE WORKOUTS:

- 20 minute row
- 4,000 meter row
- 40 seconds harder, 20 seconds easier or 15-25 minutes

Introduce longer rowing with stroke rate variation.

Do four 5-minute pieces, varying the stroke rate as follows: 20 SPM for first 2 minutes; 22 SPM for next 2 minutes; and 24 SPM for last minute. Then rest by rowing very easily for 2 minutes, before starting the next 5 minutes. Your work pace should be faster than your 10 minute pace from the last workout.

Longer steady rowing.
Two 10-minute periods with three minutes rest in between. Try to go a little faster than you did in the last session. Stroke rate 20-24.

Row 1 minute hard, 1 minute easy for a total of 20 minutes. Watch the central display for your pace.

Benchmark Row: 30 minutes, non-stop. Definitely record your total meters rowed. You should repeat this workout periodically to see how you are progressing. You can also enter it in the Concept2 Online World Ranking.

Reasons Patty and Jere recommend cross-training with rowing

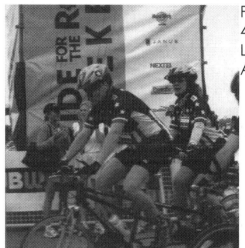

Patty and Jere at the finish line of 45 miles of the Ride for The Roses, Lance Armstrong Cancer ride in April 2002.

November 2010 Patty and Jere at finish of 26.2 mile cancer fund raising ride.

Patty and I have discovered that Indoor Rowing on the C-2 rower has improved our performance during bicycling events. Patty does not row "On The Water (OTW)". Therefore, all of Patty's rowing endurance and strength training must come from the Concept 2 Indoor rower which she uses religiously EVERY day!

The following are more reasons that rowing is an excellent add-on to any bicycling training program as cross-training :

1. Rowing exercises most muscle groups providing additional exercise and strength training to those muscle groups that are used in sports such as in cycling. This is really important to cyclists who need to maintain balance in muscle use and development. Over use and over development of muscles used in cycling only training can lead to what cyclists refer to as, "Cycling Rigor mortis".

2.Rowing offers upper AND lower body exercise. Cycling is an excellent lower body development trainer...rowing adds the upper body component.

3. Indoor rowing on the C-2 rower is a non-impact exercise. There is much less wear and tear on the body.

4. Rowing on the C-2 ERG is an indoor sport that can be done anywhere, anytime!

5. The Concept 2 Indoor Rower provides a super conditioning workout for any athletic level. The C-2 Rower has been used by the Olympics as a training tool since the Rower was invented. Because the work is self paced, old, and not so old, rowers of every ability can establish their own specific work level that will bring them success.

Workouts recommended by Concept 2 and Jere Cook C-2 Master Indoor Rowing Instructor as Cross Training on the Concept 2 Indoor Rower

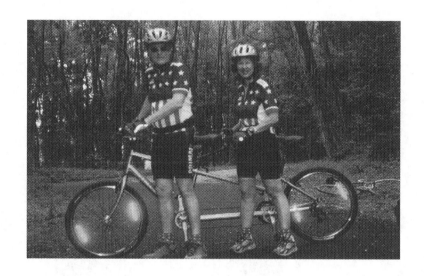

Riding Tandem in France in 2008

1. Rowing for endurance and aerobic development:

   A 30 minute row at 65 %to 75% heart rate maximum (HRM)
   10 K row at same above pace
   one hour row at same above pace

2. Rowing for strength and power development

   20 seconds hard at 80% HRM/ 40 seconds easy 70% HRM repeat 10-20 times
   30 seconds hard at 80% HRM / 1 minute easy 70% HRM repeat 10-20times

3. Rowing for intensity, speed and quickness

   500 meters at 80% HRM repeated 4-6 times with 2 min rest between
   1 minute row at 85% HRM / 1 minute row 65% HRM repeat 10-20 times

4 Rowing workout for all important recovery:

   20-40 minutes at 65% to 75% HRM
   rowing a circuit as above with implementing rowing stretches as shown in the Stretches performed on or off the C-2

Specific workouts for those who Row and Cycle or just want to be in GREAT shape

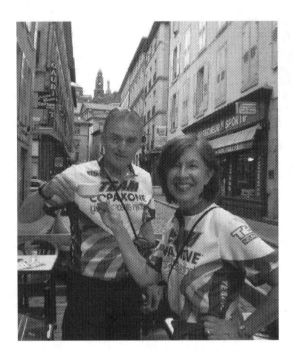

Patty and Jere celebrating with French Coffee and Chocolates in Le Puy en Velay following a ride through the French mountain sides in 2009.

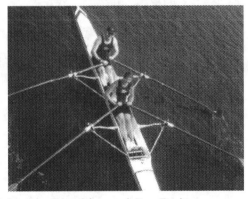

Dad (Jere Cook) and Dr. Petra (daughter) racing in recent First Coast Head Race in Jacksonville, Fl.

Patty and I have introduced many bicycle riders we ride with to using the Concept 2 Indoor Rower as a cross training routine. We recommend (as does Concept2) rowing steady pieces of between 5,000 and 10,000 meters. The workouts listed below came originally from Concept 2. As a C-2 Master Indoor Rower Instructor I recommend these pieces to my clients and our friends who are cyclists.

1. 30 minute row at a steady pace: Moderate to hard pace...60% to 80% Max Heart Rate (MHR). At each 4 minute mark row harder for 20 seconds to simulate riding hills you would normally ride. This is a great all body workout for those rainy cold days of winter.

2. 8,000 to 10,000 meter row-use a moderate pace 65% to 80% MHR. Add in the hills as above. I suggest another good way to row this piece is start slow and build to finish with a strong burst of speed.

3. One hour row- at steady state. This is especially good if you happen to have a Cycling video such as Bob Roll's CRASH video from a few years back. The video runs for one hour and takes my mind off rowing.

4. The LONG HILLY ROAD piece…this is another Concept 2 specialty piece. Warm up for 5 minutes then set the PM-3 monitor for 10,000 meters. If you are just starting to use rowing to supplement cycling training start with 5,000 meters. You can use the "Intervals" option on the PM3 and PM4 monitors to achieve this overall 10,000 or 5,000 meter row.

Row at a conversational pace, 60% to 70% MHR for 250 – 500 meters. Once you are warmed up you can increase your rowing speed and your MHR and manage both as you near the 9,000 meter point. Use the last 1,000 meters to bring your heart rate back down.

Use Stretching and Strength Training to round out an excellent training session

Follow these routines with stretching as shown in the Rowing section stretches.

Additional strength gains can be achieved by completing a few of the strength training routines using rubber bands or static exercises such as "The Plank and Side Plank" to increase your "core-strength" and stamina.

WORKOUT: BLANK FORM TO COPY

- Goal of the workout:

Description of workout: Interval workout

# of intervals	work time	intensity guide	target SPM	rest time

WARMUP: (estimated time 5 min)   Include rowing drills and on rower stretching.

WORKOUT SETUP: (estimated time min)
- Machine setup: Set Damper at 3 or other setting of choice.
- Monitor setup: Set work time for
                   Set rest time for

BODY OF WORKOUT: (estimated time _____ min)
- Remarks during workout: At each interval, increase your intensity. Try to improve your pace without increasing your strokes per minute (SPM).

Interval	Meters Rowed	Average Pace
1		
2		
3		
4		
5		
6		
7		
8		
9		
10		
Total Meters		

Cumulative Meters:

COOLDOWN: (estimated time 5 min) Include light paddling and stretching. NOTES: (estimated time 1 min)

Logging results:Use the recall button to note meters rowed and average pace for each interval.

Rowing Drills to develop technique

(see technique review in earlier section)

These drills help develop technique by focusing on one part of the stroke at a time. Allow one drill to transition into the next until a complete stroke is taken.

Arms Only: Teaches hands away before knees come up.

* Keeping legs in the finish position, row with the arms only. Knees do not move upward.

* This exercise is called the "pick drill," and it helps people learn to move "around the corner" at the catch and finish of the stroke.

* Allow the hands to float out until the arms are extended; keep the wrists relaxed.

* Be sure that the handle is pulled to within one inch of the abdomen, halfway between the lap and the chest.

Arms and Back: Demonstrates the coordinated effort of arms and back during the drive and recovery of each stroke.

* This exercise starts the same as **Arms Only**, but the handle moves past the knees as the upper body leans forward over the thighs. This demonstrates proper extension of the arms and body before the legs come up.

* Change the direction of the handle by first allowing the body to swing back.

* As the handle passes the knees, begin the arm pull as taught in **Arms Only**.

Partial Slide: Teaches proper body position and sequence at each point in the drive and recovery.

* Row each position continuously for 10 strokes; then increase the seat travel to the next position until the full slide position is reached.

* **1/4 slide** Like **Arms and Back**, but continue the extension forward with a slight bend of the knee.

- **1/2 slide** Same movement but just a little more slide. Allow the seat to come halfway up the monorail.

- **3/4 slide** Allow the seat to come 3/4 of the way up to your normal catch position. Remember to get full arm extension and pivot forward at the hips before the seat starts coming up the monorail.

- **Full slide** Row full strokes, maintaining control, and emphasize full arm extension and pivot at the hips before the seat starts coming up the monorail.

Legs Only: Teaches that the legs, not the arms and shoulders, initiate the drive.

- Start at the catch position.

- Push the legs until the handle is over the ankles (pause a second and then recover).

- Come to the catch position; then drive again.

Legs and Back: An extension of the Legs Only drill.

- Start at the catch position.

- Push the legs and pivot at the hips but leave the arms straight..

- Begin the move to the catch position by first pivoting forward at the hips and then moving the seat up the monorail with your legs. The arms remain straight.

- Feel the pressure you can generate without pulling in with their arms.

Ultra-Slow-Motion Rowing: Gets all of the body parts working in the right order.

- Row as low as 10 strokes per minute (SPM).

- Work on being very deliberate and getting the proper sequence on the recovery and the drive.

Recommended Stretches—for Before and After Rowing

STRETCHES PERFORMED ON OR USING THE INDOOR ROWER

These stretches can be incorporated into the warmup and cooldown for all workouts. We suggest that you try all these stretches and develop a routine using the stretches that work best for you.

Before Stretching: row lightly for 3-5 minutes to get the blood flowing and begin to warm up the body.

Pre-Workout Stretches can be held for approximately 10 seconds.

Post-Workout Stretches can be held for up to 30 seconds.

All Stretches:
• should be done in a static, relaxed and patient fashion. NO bouncing or abrupt movements.

• should include full deep breaths, expanding the diaphragm on inhalation, for maximum results.

• should be repeated on both sides if a unilateral stretch.

• can be repeated for 3-5 repetitions.

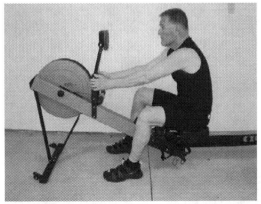

1. Posterior deltoids, Lattissimus Dorsi. Trapezius, Scapulae Musculature

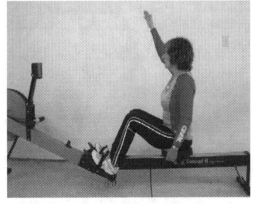

2. Obliques, Latissimus Dorsi

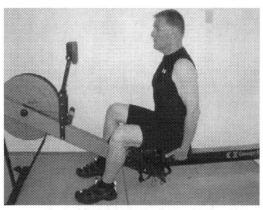

3. Anterior Deltoids, Rectus Abdominis

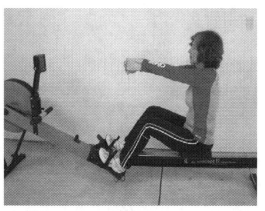

4. Biceps

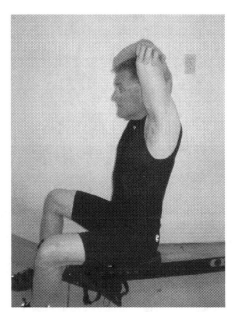

5. Triceps

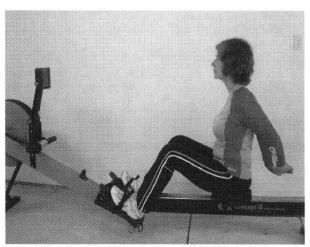

6. Anterior Deltoids, Pectoralis Major and Minor

Continue stretches on the Indoor Rower:

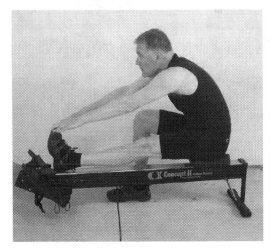

7. Hamstrings

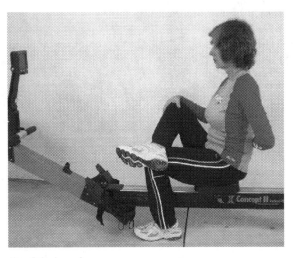

8. Gluteals

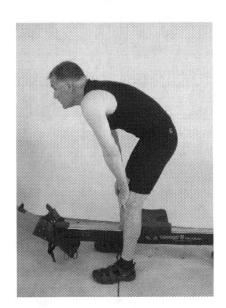

9. Lumbar region, Erector Spinae

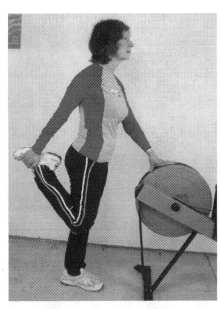

10. Quadriceps, Hip Flexors

Stretches for rowing without using the Indoor Rower
Part I

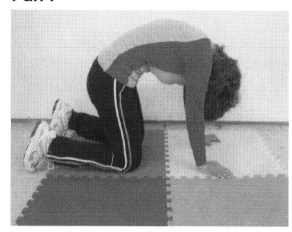

Lumbar and Thoracic Regions

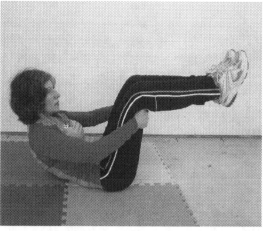

Lumbar and Thoracic on back

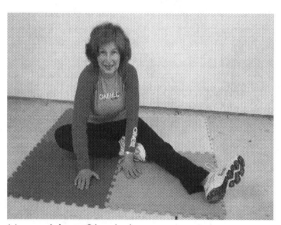

Hamstring Stretch

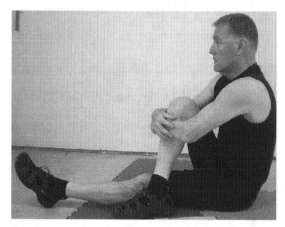

Gluteus

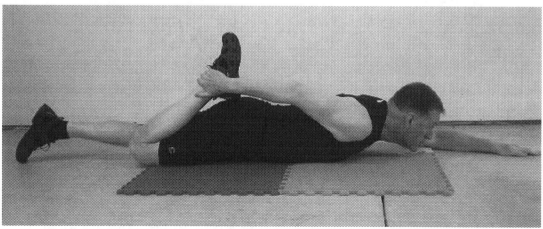

Quadriceps, Hip Flexors

Stretches for rowing without using the Indoor Rower
Part II

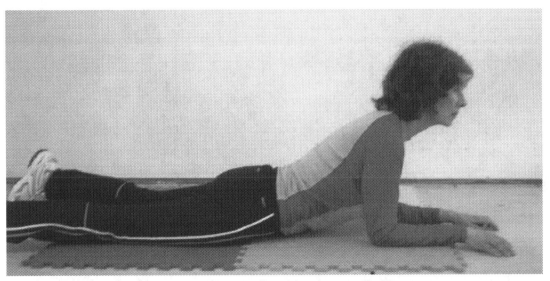

Rectus Abdominus

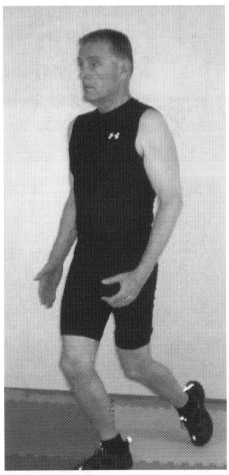

Tibialis Anterior

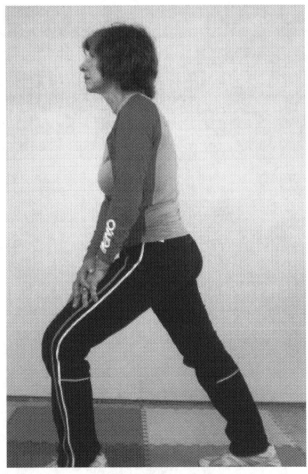

Gastrocnemius, Achilles Region

Bicycling Training

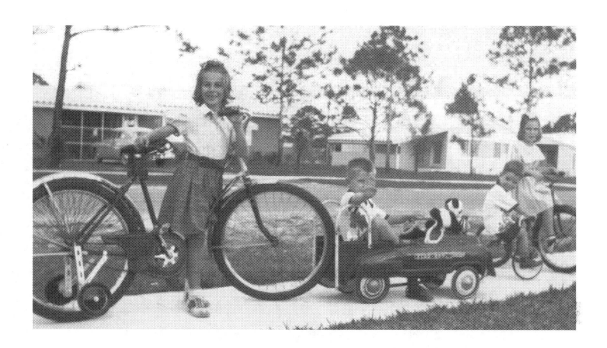

◊   Bicycling for Fitness and Fun

◊   Bicycle Warm-up Cool Down & Stretching

◊   Bicycle Strength Training

◊   Bicycle Endurance Rides to Build Endurance

BICYCLING for FITNESS and FUN

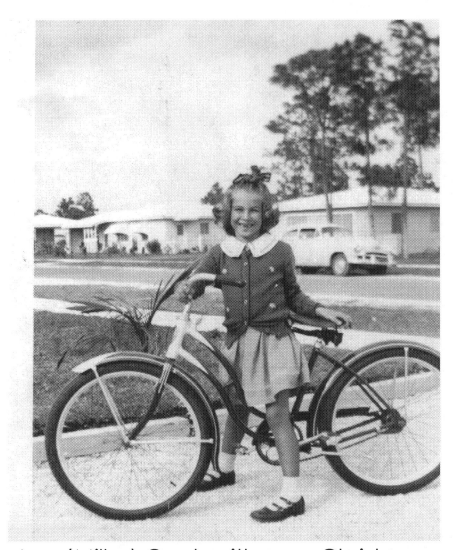

Patty Ann (Miller) Cook with new Christmas bicycle

Bicycling is for everyone and anyone who wants fitness, relaxation and fun. In early 2009, post economic melt-down, bicycling has enjoyed an enormous return to popularity. On any day millions of people can be found riding for fun and now for economic reasons. As with all the exercise options discussed herein, Patty and I recommend you know your **safe heart rate range**, and use a heart rate monitor to regulate and manage your exercise to keep you in a strength building but safe zone.

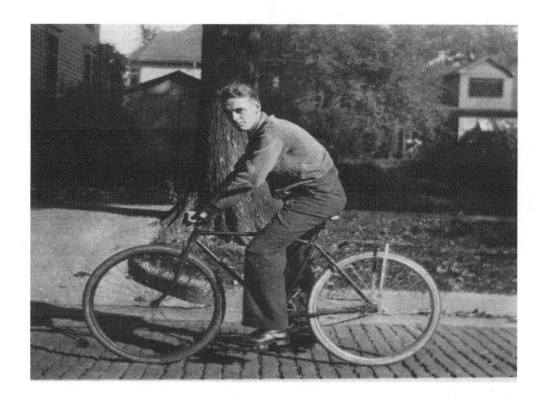

Gerard Cook, age 19, 1934 University of Illinois student (Jere's father and Petra's grandfather)

Patty and I have always ridden bicycles. When we were growing up our parents bought us bicycles and encouraged us to ride. Early in our marriage I would ride during triathlons and Patty and Petra would cheer me on. We all had single bicycles and rode together, or alone, often.

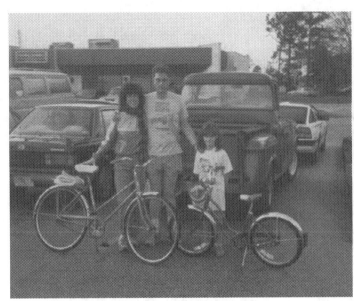

Patty, Petra and Jere at ½ Marathon 1985 (Petra was 5 years old!)

Patty and Petra rode their bicycles 13.5 miles with me running the Jacksonville Thanksgiving 1/2 Marathon in 1985.

In the early 1990's we bought our tandem bicycle. From the moment we bought it we knew we had a winner.

Ride for the Roses, with Lance Armstrong 2002, Patty and Jere at start.

Jere was diagnosed with melanoma cancer two months after this ride.

We have ridden our tandem in Texas with Lance Armstrong in the Ride for the Roses ® and many other rides around the USA. Our Tandem rides have been in California, Vermont (killer

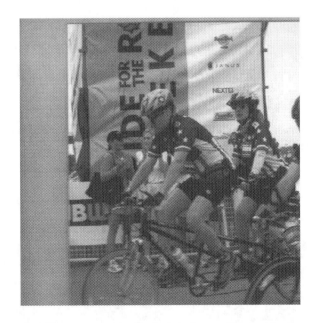

mountains), Washington State (BIGGER killer mountains), Maine, Georgia (Tour of Georgia) and all around Florida. We have also ridden Tandem bicycles in England, Ireland (Dublin – Galway) and France.

Tandem bicycles have been referred to as marriage "Makers and Breakers". If you chose to ride tandem Patty and I encourage you to talk to each other constantly. Neither of you are totally "in charge". The Captain up front steers the ship while the back-seat tail gunner known as the "Stoker" controls the power input and balance. Tandems are really great. Since we purchased our tandem we have logged over 10,000 miles on it. Amazing! Bicycling IS an excellent way to exercise, stay in great shape, have fun, meet many very interesting people and see great scenery.

For the completion of my Masters Degree Thesis, I used data from the US Air Force (National Guard) bicycling team I formed. This team was composed of US Air Force and civilian personnel. Our goal was for the riders (men and women) to train and ride in, and complete, the 1998 Multiple Sclerosis 150 mile Charity Ride (MS-150). My Thesis was a success, the bicycle team raised thousands of dollars for MS and the team photo was placed on the cover of the National Guard magazine.

In my studies I learned many things that Patty and I use today to help keep us flexible, in shape and riding often 4 times a week! The Cooper Institute for Aerobic Research (CIAR) and in articles from the American College of Sports Medicine (ACSM) I learned that aerobic exercise researchers have established that 20 to 60 minutes a day, 3 to 5 days per week is excellent for toning large muscles of the upper and lower body. The cycling also boosts cardiovascular strength without the damaging stress of running. ACSM and CIAR physicians advise older adults and people with joint problems to cycle, thereby reducing stress on joints and muscles.

Cycling works primarily the muscles in the legs, hips, buttocks and the muscles in the body core; an added plus is that the oxidative capacity of the body is also improved. Most importantly the myocardial muscle, the heart, is given as strong a workout as desired. Patty and I recommend you obtain one of the many "heart-rate training" books on the market and use the book and heart-rate monitor to begin your weight loss + strength, training while riding your bicycle.

Bicycle Warm-up, Cool Down & Stretching

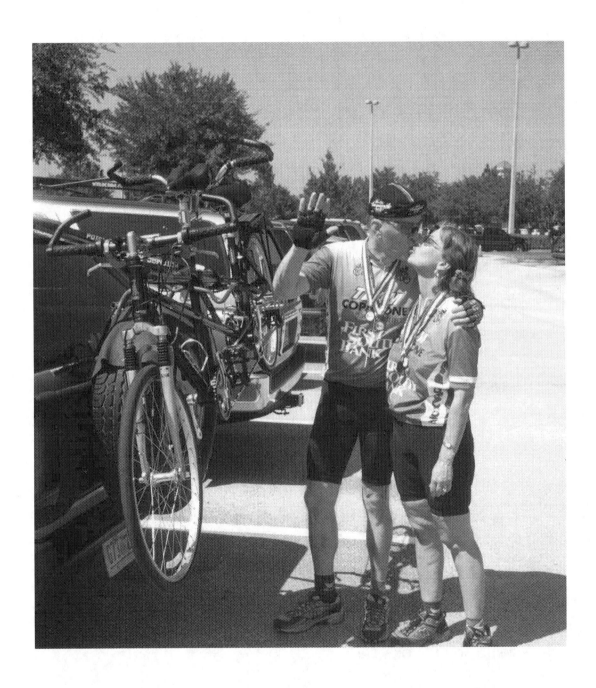

BICYCLING: WARM-UP; COOL DOWN; + STRETCH

One of the most appealing things about bicycling to Patty and me is that bicycling is pretty easy on our bodies. We enjoy peddling because there is no pounding, no twisting, no extreme ranges of motion (except for me on my road racing bicycle in the "egg" shape). Patty especially enjoys bicycling because all she needs to do is sit and pedal and watch the calories disappear while the muscles firm up.

Many people never have and probably never will consider warming up, cooling down or stretching any time before, during or after riding. We hope you will read our suggestions and begin a routine of warm-up, stretching and cool down when ever you ride.

As with all our sports, we recommend you develop the good habit of warming up prior to beginning an exercise session. The good reasons for warming up have been stated elsewhere in this book, however, we will mention them again specifically for bicycling.

The best way to warm-up prior to a bicycle training ride of any length is, "RIDE YOUR BICYCLE"! As your body warms up your muscles contract quicker as oxygen is delivered easily to the muscles of your legs, body core and even arms. Patty especially enjoys the idea of melting off pounds as her heart rate increases and she burns calories.

As you warm up your body cycling, your heart rate will increase. Use either the Rate of Perceived Exertion (RPE) or a heart rate monitor to help you control your level of effort. Build your heart rate up gradually. You will know you are starting to warm up when you begin to start to sweat. You can consider yourself "warmed-up" when your heart rate is about 60% to 70% of your heart rate maximum. Once you are warmed up it may be a good time to stop and perform the stretches shown later in this section.

Remember that stretching when the muscles are not warmed up could be counter-productive to your exercise efforts and may cause unnecessary pain or injury. In the section on stretching, we discovered the science facts about stretching. Now it is time to visually see some of the most recommended stretches for bicyclists.

What we discovered about the most recent research about stretching indicates that stretching will not hurt your exercise experience and may actually help you stay more flexible and injury free. Warm-up is necessary and slow, relaxed stretches seem to work best. Patty and I strongly recommend that you do NOT bounce your body while stretching. Try to hold each stretch for 20 to 30 seconds. We try to visualize blood rushing into the muscle as flexibility increases.

Patty is as flexible as a 17 year old girl...she is lucky. Meanwhile, at my 62 years old, with many military deployments to very cold and very warm environments along with a lifetime of physical activity, I feel "bicycle rigor mortis" setting into my body following each ride! That is the reason I stretch.

I stretch so I can ride, walk and row another day. Patty stretches because it feels good and she knows it is good for her joints and ligaments. So here are some of our most used stretches performed after warm-up, when we stop for coffee break or snacks, and especially following each ride.

BICYCLING SPECIFIC STRETCHES

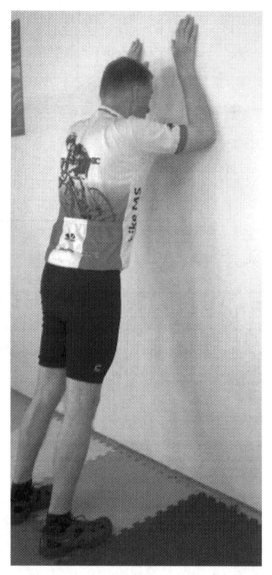

ACHILLES TENDON + CALF MUSCLE STRETCH

Stand about 2 feet away from any vertical surface: in this photo I am standing facing a wall with my feet flat on the floor, palms against the flat surface and above my head. Lean forward until your elbows touch the wall. Feel for the stretch in your heels and along the lower back of your leg. These areas can become very tight following long rides with little stretching.

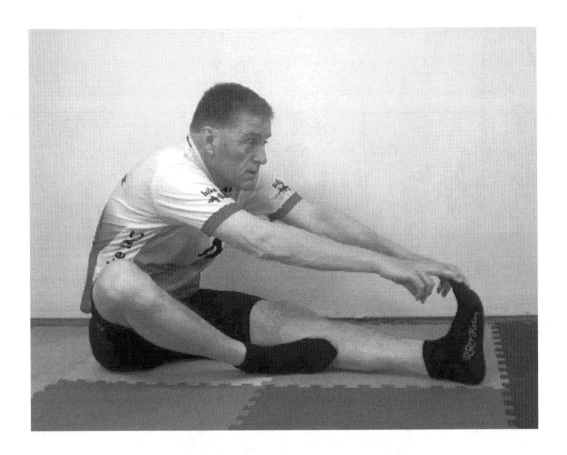

HAMSTRINGS STRETCH / MODIFIED

This stretch can be done sitting on the ground or standing up with your heel resting on an object at about waist height. In this case I am sitting on the ground with one leg stretched out in front of me. In this photo my left leg is outstretched while my right heel is brought toward my crotch. My heel goes against my thigh making a 90 degree angle. While I keep my left leg straight I bend at my waist, slowly lowering my body toward my left thigh while slowly reaching out toward my left toes. Feel the stretch along the back of the left thigh and leg in general. Well stretched ham string muscles can greatly reduce back pain due to too tight hamstrings.

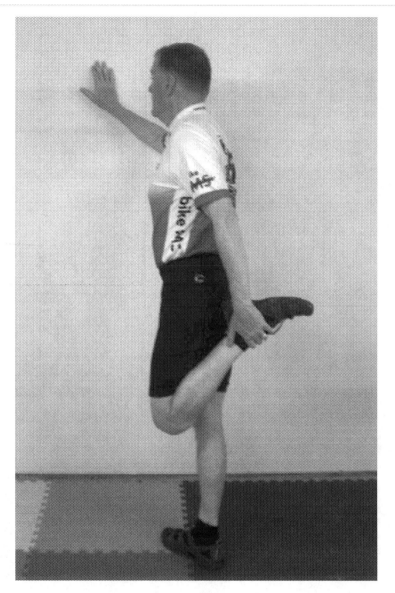

STRETCH FOR QUADRICEPS, CAN BE DONE LAYING DOWN

Good stretch for front of leg. Not recommended if you are experiencing knee pain or knee joint problems. Stand as shown and reach behind you. You may have to bend you straight leg to reach your ankle. Pull your leg toward your buttocks. Pull only to the point where you feel tension and a stretch in your muscles. DO NOT over stretch.

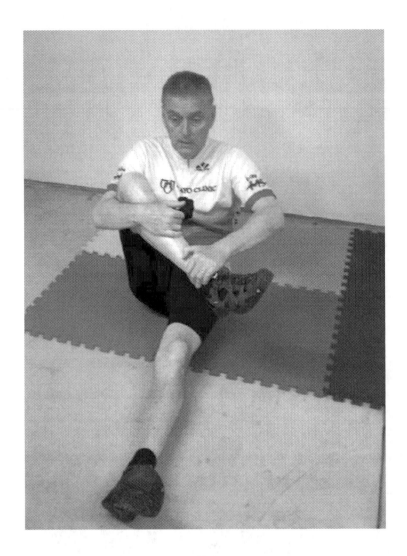

STRETCH FOR HIPS AND BUTTOCKS

This stretch may also be accomplished while standing. It is easier to perform if you are sitting on the ground. You will see a similar stretch in the Rowing Stretches section. You may use either or both stretches for cycling and/or rowing.

Sit on the floor and bend one knee as you slide the ankle toward your midsection. Grasp your ankle with one hand while you hook your elbow around your knee for support. Gently pull your foot toward your opposite shoulder. Feel for the stretch in your buttocks (piriformis and gluteus)

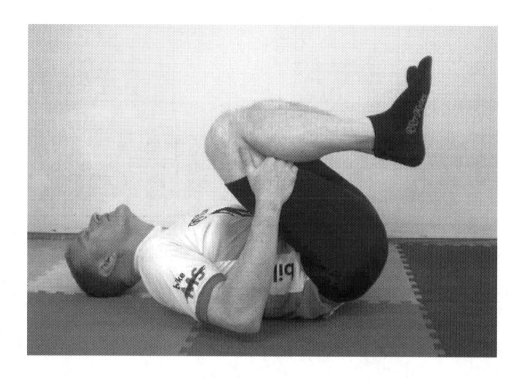

STRETCH FOR LOWER BACK TO RELAX MUSCLES

This is a must do stretch if you plan to ride long distances or for long periods of time. Stop as often as you wish. Lie on your back and bend your knees toward your chin. Reach down and grasp your legs behind your thighs. Try to keep your head on the ground. Pull your knees toward your chest until your hips come up off the ground. I recommend you hold this stretch, as well as all stretches, for 20 to 30 seconds for maximum benefit. Feel the stretch in your lower back. SLOWLY extend one leg, then the other and roll to one side to stand up.

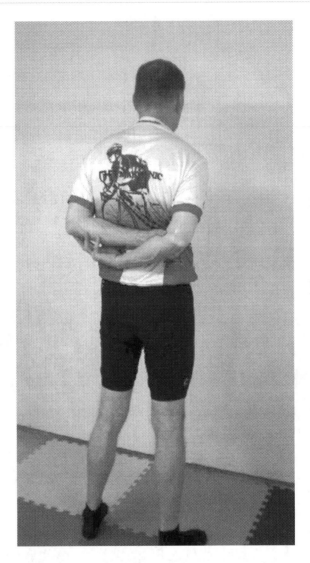

STRETCH FOR SHOULDERS AND NECK

When I first started to perform this stretch about 30 years ago I was so tight that I could barely get my hands to touch behind my back...I could not move my hands anywhere near my elbows. What a difference now from then!

Stand as shown with both arms behind back. Reach to grasp your left elbow with your right hand or as near as you can get for now...do not try to reach too far if you are not flexible enough now...you will improve over time. Pull your elbow across your body mid-section toward the right while tilting your head toward your right shoulder. Move only your head, try to not tilt at waist. Reverse sides and repeat.

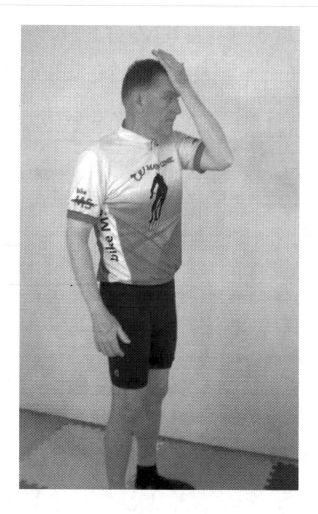

STRETCH FOR NECK AND SHOULDERS

If you ride Road Bikes or even Mountain Bikes for any length of time you will discover that your neck will become stiff from holding your head up to see where you are going. Years ago I watched the Japanese Air Force Officers I rode with in Misawa, Japan do this stretch. It helped my neck then and it still does today.

Stand up straight. Place one hand on your forehead and the other at your side. Press your forehead gently forward into the palm of your hand as you resist your head moving forward. You should feel pressure all around your neck and shoulders. Hold the pressure for 20 to 30 seconds or as long as you feel comfortable. When you release the pressure you should feel your neck and shoulders relax. I hope this works as well for you as it does for me.

Strength Training For Cycling

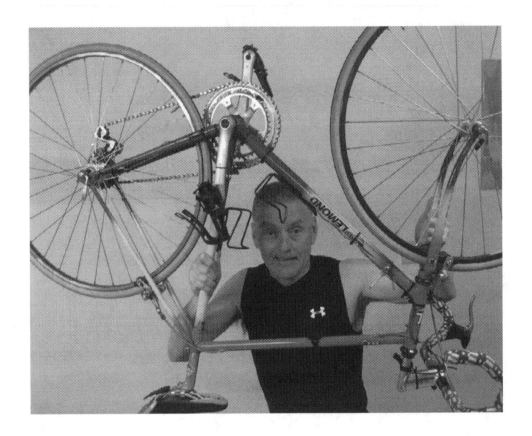

Follow Strength Training
General Plan
In This Book.

Bicycle Endurance Rides to Build Endurance

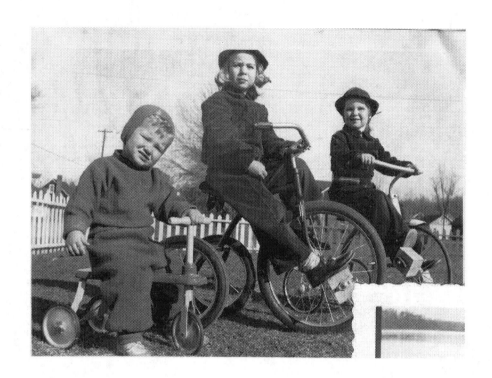

◊   SAMPLE RIDES FROM JERE AND PATTY.

◊   4 RIDES FROM PATTY

◊   10 RIDES FROM JERE

◊   BLANK FORM TO MAKE YOUR OWN RIDE

◊   SAMPLE SCHEDULE FOR ONE WEEK OF RIDES

PATTY'S CHOICE OF GOOD PRACTICE RIDES

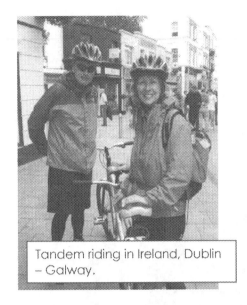

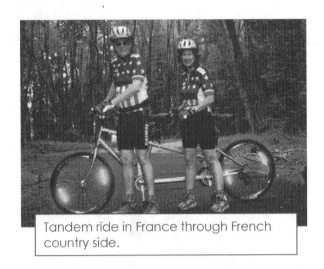

Tandem ride in France through French country side.

Tandem riding in Ireland, Dublin – Galway.

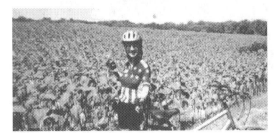

Patty in sun flower field just like Tour de France.

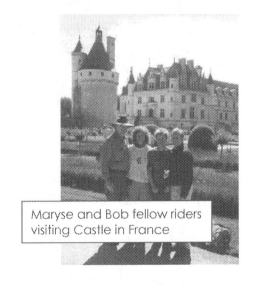

Maryse and Bob fellow riders visiting Castle in France

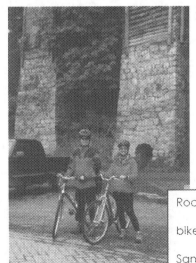

Roche Harbor Lime Kilns part of 45 mile

bike ride in cold rain

San Juan Island, 2008.

PATTY'S CHOICE OF GOOD PRACTICE RIDES

RIDE # 1 FLAT ROAD (Patricia's House Ride).

TOTAL TIME: About 40 MINUTES

WARM-UP: 5 minutes easy pedaling in a small gear at 70 to 80 RPM; it is ok to stop at end of warm-up ride to stretch.

Distance: 10 miles: 5 miles out and 5 miles return

Speed: will vary in miles per hour based on grade of hill

Time: 20 - 35 minutes +/-

Terrain: Flat Road through beautiful old homes with many flowers

Pace: Steady, shift as required to keep workload feeling constant. Maintain   cadence of 70 to 75 RPM as best possible.

Effort: 60% to 70% of Heart Rate Maximum (HRM). Slow down as needed to control heart rate.

Cool Down: At ride end, 5 minutes easy pedaling 60 to 65 RPM...then stretch (see stretches).

Estimated Possible Calories Burned: 31 calories per mile depending on your effort.

Good beginners ride. Nice ride through beautiful residential area on way to one of our favorite coffee shops in Jacksonville.

Endurance - Bicycling

PATTY'S CHOICE OF GOOD PRACTICE RIDES

RIDE # 2 FLAT ROAD (River Road Ride).

TOTAL TIME: About 55 to 60 MINUTES

WARM-UP: 5 minutes easy pedaling in a small gear at 70 to 80 RPM it is ok to stop at end of warm-up ride to stretch.

Distance: 12 to 13 miles: large loop along beautiful St. Johns River. Can be extremely windy...similar to riding up steep hill.

Speed: will vary in miles per hour based on grade of hill and speed and direction of wind

Time: 55 to 60 minutes +/-

Terrain: Generally flat road with 2 small hills. The wind along the river for 2.5 miles can be difficult...watch your heart rate closely.

Pace: Steady, shift as required to keep workload feeling constant. Maintain cadence of 70 to 75 RPM as best possible.

Effort: 60% to 70% of Heart Rate Maximum (HRM). Slow down as needed to control heart rate.

Cool Down: At ride end, 5 minutes easy pedaling 60 to 65 RPM...then stretch (see stretches).

Estimated Possible Calories Burned: 31 calories per mile depending on your effort.

PATTY'S CHOICE OF GOOD PRACTICE RIDES

RIDE # 3 Flat Paved Trail loop with steep bridge in middle .

TOTAL TIME: About 60 to 90 MINUTES

(Jere and I rode this route often using the bridge as training for our mountain rides in Washington State in 2008.)

WARM-UP: 5 minutes easy pedaling in a small gear at 70 to 90 RPM it is ok to stop at end of warm-up ride to stretch.

Distance: 17 to 21 miles: large loop on Black Creek bicycle trail, Clay County, Fl..

Speed: will vary in miles per hour based on grade of hill and speed and direction of wind

Time: 60 to 90 minutes +/-

Terrain: Generally flat paved trail with very steep bridge in middle. Wind can be a problem.

Pace: Steady, shift as required to keep workload feeling constant. Maintain cadence of 75 to 85 RPM as best possible.

Effort: 65% to 85% of Heart Rate Maximum (HRM). Slow down as needed to control heart rate.

Cool Down: At ride end, 5 minutes easy pedaling 60 to 65 RPM...then stretch (see stretches).

Estimated Possible Calories Burned: 35 calories per mile depending on your effort.

Endurance - Bicycling

PATTY'S CHOICE OF GOOD PRACTICE RIDES

RIDE # 4 Rolling Paved Trail loop with several steep bridges in middle.

TOTAL TIME: About 70 to 100 MINUTES

(Jere and I rode this route often using the bridges as training for our mountain rides in Washington State in 2008.)

WARM-UP: 5 minutes easy pedaling in a small gear at 70 to 90 RPM it is ok to stop at end of warm-up ride to stretch.

Distance: 22 to 30 miles: large loop from near NAS JAX Naval Air Station to downtown Jacksonville with stops at two coffee shops as needed.

Speed: will vary in miles per hour based on grade of hills and speed and direction of wind

Time: 70 to 100 minutes +/-

Terrain: Rolling paved trail with very steep bridges in middle. Wind can be a problem.

Pace: Variable, shift as required to keep workload feeling constant. Maintain cadence of 75 to 85 RPM as best possible. Ride 5 minutes at 70% to 75% HRM, then ride 75% to 85% HRM for 10 minutes. Repeat this sequence 5 times if possible.

Effort: 65% to 85% of Heart Rate Maximum (HRM). Slow down as needed to control heart rate.

Cool Down: At ride end, 5 minutes easy pedaling 60 to 65 RPM...then stretch (see stretches).

Estimated Possible Calories Burned: 30-35 calories per mile depending on your effort.

JERE'S CHOICE OF GOOD PRACTICE RIDES

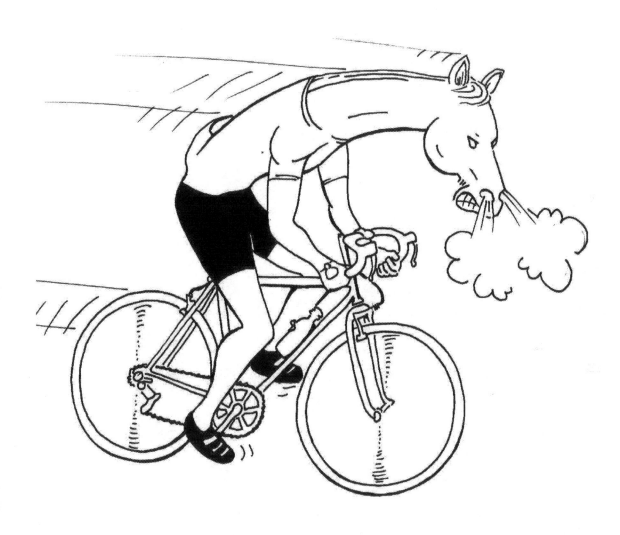

Endurance - Bicycling

EXAMPLE RIDES

RIDE # 1 Just Starting / or any easy ride.

TOTAL TIME: About 30 to 40 MINUTES

WARM-UP: 5 to 7 minutes easy pedaling in a small gear at 60 to 70 RPM; it is ok to stop at end of warm-up ride to stretch.

Distance: 3 - 5 miles

Speed: 10 to 11 mile per hour

Time: 20 - 30 minutes +/-

Terrain: Flat road

Pace: Steady, shift as required to keep workload feeling constant. Maintain cadence of 70 to 75 RPM.

Effort: 60% to 70% of Heart Rate Maximum (HRM). Slow down as needed to control heart rate.

Cool Down: At ride end, 5 to 7 minutes easy pedaling 60 to 70 RPM...then stretch (see stretches).

Estimated Possible Calories Burned: About 30 calories per mile.

If this is your 1st ride on a new bicycle, get accustomed to the bicycle by moving your hands around on the handle bars, practice shifting and braking and get comfortable with stopping and starting.

EXAMPLE RIDES

RIDE # 2 Training Ride.

TOTAL TIME: About 30 to 40 MINUTES

WARM-UP: 5 to 7 minutes easy pedaling in a small gear at 60 to 70 RPM; it is ok to stop at end of warm-up ride to stretch.

Distance: 3 - 6 miles

Speed: 10 to 11 mile per hour

Time: 30 - 40 minutes +/-

Terrain: Flat road

Pace: Steady, shift as required to keep workload feeling constant. Maintain cadence of 70 to 75 RPM.

Effort: 65% to 70% of Heart Rate Maximum (HRM). Slow down as needed to control heart rate.

Cool Down: At ride end, 5 to 7 minutes easy pedaling 60 to 75 RPM...then stretch (see stretches).

Estimated Possible Calories Burned: About 31 calories per mile.

_____

Endurance - Bicycling

EXAMPLE RIDES

RIDE # 3 Training Ride.

TOTAL TIME: About 35 to 40 MINUTES

WARM-UP: 5 to 7 minutes easy pedaling in a small gear at 65 to 75 RPM; it is ok to stop at end of warm-up ride to stretch.

Distance: 9 miles

Speed: 11 to 13 mile per hour

Time: 40 minutes +/-

Terrain: Flat road

Pace: Steady, shift as required to keep workload feeling constant. Maintain cadence of 75 to 79 RPM.

Effort: 65% to 75% of Heart Rate Maximum (HRM). Slow down as needed to control heart rate.

Cool Down: At ride end, 5 to 7 minutes easy pedaling 65 to 70 RPM…then stretch (see stretches).

Estimated Possible Calories Burned: About 31 calories per mile.

Good midweek ride for beginners or "an active rest"

EXAMPLE RIDES

RIDE # 4 Rolling Hills .

TOTAL TIME: About 40 to 45 MINUTES

WARM-UP: 9 - 10 minutes easy pedaling in a small gear at 70 to 80 RPM; it is ok to stop at end of warm-up ride to stretch.

Distance: 6 miles

Speed: will vary in miles per hour based on grade of hill

Time: 30 - 35 minutes +/-

Terrain: Gentle rolling hills

Pace: Steady, shift as required to keep workload feeling constant. Maintain cadence of 70 to 75 RPM.

Effort: 60% to 70% of Heart Rate Maximum (HRM). Slow down as needed to control heart rate.

Cool Down: At ride end, 5 minutes easy pedaling 70 to 75 RPM...then stretch (see stretches).

Estimated Possible Calories Burned: 35 - 40 calories per mile depending on your effort.

Good beginners ride for those want to extend their fitness through the adaptation principle of mild increased stress on cardio – muscle system. Also good for fit cyclist who wants to maintain fitness level.

Endurance - Bicycling

EXAMPLE RIDES

RIDE # 5 Rolling Hills .

TOTAL TIME: About 40 to 45 MINUTES

WARM-UP: 10 minutes easy pedaling in a small gear at 80 RPM; it is ok to stop at end of warm-up ride to stretch.

Distance: 7 miles

Speed: will vary in miles per hour based on grade of hill

Time: 45 minutes +/-

Terrain: Rolling hills

Pace: Steady, shift as required to keep workload feeling constant. Maintain cadence of 70 to 80 RPM.

Effort: 70% to 80% of Heart Rate Maximum (HRM). Slow down as needed to control heart rate.

Cool Down: At ride end, 5 minutes easy pedaling   85 RPM…then stretch (see stretches).

Estimated Possible Calories Burned: 30 - 40 calories per mile depending on your effort.

Good beginners ride for those want to extend their fitness through the adaptation principle of mild increased stress on cardio – muscle system. Ride is good for fit cyclist who wants to maintain fitness level.

EXAMPLE RIDES

RIDE # 6 Stationary Bike Ride on adjustable resistance .

TOTAL TIME: About 40 to 45 MINUTES

WARM-UP: 6 minutes easy pedaling in a small gear with light resistance at 85 - 90 RPM; it is ok to stop at end of warm-up ride to stretch.

Distance: To be Determined (TBD)

Time: 35 minutes +/-

Terrain:

Pace: Light resistance for 10 minutes then adjust for moderate resistance for 25 minutes; cadence of 75 to 85 rpm.

Effort: 65% to 70% of Heart Rate Maximum (HRM). Slow down as needed to control heart rate.

Cool Down: At ride end, 5 minutes easy pedaling 0 resistance   85 RPM… then stretch (see stretches).

Estimated Possible Calories Burned: 7 – 8 calories per min depending on your effort.

Good beginners ride for those want to extend their fitness through the adaptation principle of mild increased stress on cardio – muscle system. Ride is good for fit cyclist who wants to maintain fitness level. Important to maintain recommended RPM.

EXAMPLE RIDES

RIDE #7 Heart Rate Training ride with Variable Intensity .

TOTAL TIME: About 1 hour +/-

WARM-UP: 10 minutes easy pedaling in a small gear at 85 - 90 RPM; it is ok to stop at end of warm-up ride to stretch.

Distance: 14 miles

Time: 60 to 75 minutes +/-

Terrain: Flat or very low rolling hills.

Pace: HEART RATE training ride: 30 minutes at 60 – 65% HRMax, then 20 minutes at 65 – 85% HRMax, then cool down to 60%, cadence of 75 to 90 rpm. Use HR and speed to finish the 14 miles safely.

Effort: 60% to 85% of Heart Rate Maximum (HRM). Slow down as needed to   control heart rate.

Cool Down: At ride end, 5 minutes easy pedaling   85 RPM…then stretch (see   stretches).

Estimated Possible Calories Burned: 7 – 15 calories per min depending on your   effort.

Good ride for those who want to extend their fitness through the adaptation principle of mild increased stress on cardio + muscle system.

EXAMPLE RIDES

RIDE #8 Gradual Hill: Heart Rate Training Ride

(Patty and I used this to get ready to ride hills on San Juan Island, Wash., 2008).

TOTAL TIME: About 1 hour +/-

WARM-UP: 10 minutes easy pedaling in a small gear at 85 - 90 RPM. It is ok to stop at end of warm-up ride to stretch.

Distance: 7 - 8 miles

Time: 45 - 65 minutes +/- ride to heart rate

Terrain: Gradual hill.

Pace: HEART RATE training ride: 22 minutes at 60 – 75% HRMax, then 30 minutes at 65 – 80% HRM, then cool down to 60% HRM, cadence of 75 to 90 rpm. Use HR and speed to finish the hill climb safely.

Effort: 60% to 80% of Heart Rate Maximum (HRM). Slow down as needed to control heart rate.

Cool Down: At ride end, 5 minutes easy pedaling 0 resistance   85 RPM… then   stretch (see stretches).

Estimated Possible Calories Burned: 30 to 45 calories per mile depending on your effort.

Professional riders know to "lift up their legs when riding up hills". You can do this with simple toe clips like the ones on police mountain bikes. When going up any hill, sit up straight and lift legs up with gluteus, quadriceps and hamstrings in your legs.

EXAMPLE RIDES

RIDE # 9 Flat or Rolling Hills .

TOTAL TIME: About 40 to 45 MINUTES

WARM-UP: 10 minutes easy pedaling in a small gear at 80 RPM it is ok to stop at end of warm-up ride to stretch.

Distance: 7 miles

Speed: will vary in miles per hour based on grade of hill

Time: 45 minutes +/-

Terrain: Rolling hills

Pace: Steady, shift as required to keep workload feeling constant. Maintain cadence of 70 to 80 RPM.

Effort: 70% to 80% of Heart Rate Maximum (HRM). Slow down as needed to control heart rate.

Cool Down: At ride end, 5 minutes easy pedaling   85 RPM…then stretch (see stretches).

Estimated Possible Calories Burned: 30 - 40 calories per mile depending on your effort.

Good beginners ride for those want to extend their fitness through the adaptation principle of mild increased stress on cardio – muscle system. Ride is good for fit cyclist who wants to maintain fitness level.

EXAMPLE RIDES

RIDE # 10 Flat

TOTAL TIME: 75 to 90 MINUTES +/-

WARM-UP: 10 minutes easy pedaling in a small gear at 80 RPM; it is ok to stop at end of warm-up ride to stretch.

Distance: 25 miles

Speed: will vary in miles per hour based on grade of any hill

Time: 75 to 90 minutes +/-

Terrain: Flat

Pace: Variable, This is another great heart rate training ride. Ride 5 minutes at 70%-75 % HRM. Continue ride for 10 minutes at 60% to 75% HRM. Repeat sequence 4 times or more depending on your level of fitness. Try to maintain RPM 80-90.

Effort: 60% to 85% HRM Slow down as needed to control heart rate.

Cool Down: At ride end, 5 minutes easy pedaling   85 RPM...then stretch (see stretches).

Estimated Possible Calories Burned: 35 - 50 calories per mile depending on your effort.

This ride is another good ride to extend fitness through the adaptation principle of increased stress on cardio – muscle system. Ride is also good for fit cyclist who wants to maintain fitness level.

Endurance - Bicycling

EXAMPLE RIDES: BLANK – FORM   (COPY AND REUSE)

RIDE # .

TOTAL TIME: MINUTES +/-

WARM-UP:

Distance: miles

Speed:

Time: minutes +/-

Terrain:

Pace: Variable

% HRM.

Bicycle RPM .

Effort: % HRM Slow down as needed to control heart rate.

Cool Down: At ride end, 5 minutes easy pedaling   85 RPM...then stretch (see stretches).

Estimated Possible Calories Burned: calories per mile depending on your effort.

Comments about this ride:

ONE WEEK OF TRAINING RIDES

SUN	MON	TUE	WED	THUR	FRI	SAT
JERE RIDE #1	REST	PATTY RIDE #1	REST	JERE RIDE #2	REST	PATTY RIDE #3

Strength Training

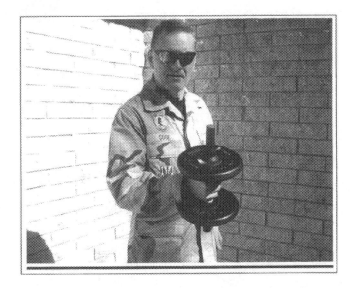

STAY IN SHAPE

Colonel Jere Cook, RED HORSE (full Colonel-06)
Commander:

Cover of a Stay In Shape Pamphlet I printed for
my squadron Advance Party as we prepared
to deploy to Iraq in Dec 2002. We all departed
safely and returned safely.

"As we age, gravity damage becomes more evident on our bodies.
Gravity damage is seen in our posture or gait and the overall way we
move and function. A good resistance training program carried on
through out life can make a difference in lessening the negative effects of
gravity."

AGE Defying Element RESISTANCE (Strength) TRAINING

Resistance training consists of relatively short bursts of muscular force anywhere between 1 second and 2 minutes. Known also as strength training, resistance training can play a part in battling certain diseases such as diabetes, arthritis, high blood pressure and prevention of osteoporosis because resistance training strengthens the body's bone density. A good strength training program carried on throughout your life can make the difference in how we are affected by gravity. This gravity defying fact alone should make every baby-boomer start a weight loss and resistance / weight lifting program immediately! Cosmetically, strength training builds shapes and even sculpts the human body like nothing else.

Resistance training develops the muscles that give shape to the body. In addition, due to the metabolic increase associated with lean muscle tissue, strength/resistance training is one key to reducing body fat.

The body stores energy in muscles for immediate use in an explosive force mode. One to two days per week of strength training is a maintenance routine with little change in strength. Three days or more bring about physiological changes...remember it is very important NOT to repeat the same routine of strength training day after day. Your body will quickly tell you why this is a bad idea with sore muscles and sore joints. Perform upper body work one day then lower body work the next day. I use our home exercise equipment and the nearby U. S. Navy military gym for my strength training, usually for 30 minutes to one hour. A schedule of 3 to 5 times a week should work well. At The Cooper Institute we learned the importance of performing some sort of exercise every day...just not the same ones every day.

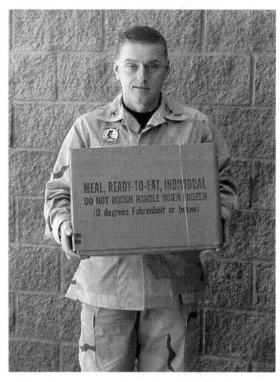

"MRE's: the troops may not eat them...but they do lift the full cases for exercise".

Sergeant Tilley's comment when he caught me lifting MRE cases.

During my many military deployments over 35+ years in the Air Force, I quickly discovered there were no gyms in many of the third world places I was deployed. To solve the challenge of strength training without hard iron weights or machines, I turned to push-ups, abdominal crunches, lifting rocks and other heavy objects (automobile transmissions, MRE cases) ... AND using rubber band technology.

Since 1975 to today when I make business trips, now as a military consultant, I always carry my "GYM IN A BAG". Patty and I both bring our carry bag "gym" on all our travels. You will see many of the types of (Dynamic Progressive Resistance) rubber bands available in the photos in this book. I suggest that you go to www.power-systems.com or any other fitness equipment supplier to find a host of portable elastic exercise equipment.

You will also see that my strength routines in this manual are completed almost entirely using elastic band technology. I use the rubber bands routinely so that I can always perform any routine I wish...and so I can NOT talk myself out of exercising because I can not find a gym.

Strength

You need to know these terms to follow along on some of the strength exercises later in this section.

Reps (repetitions, 1-2-3-4-5...etc) and Sets (set of repetitions performed in one time period of exercise). Perform one arm curl 10 times and stop... that is 10 reps in one set.

The following are a few general tips from the world of Personal Trainers:

1. Start slowly with one or two sets of 5 to 7 repetitions per set at low to moderate resistance.

2. After 1 to 2 weeks increase the sets to 3 or 4 and the repetitions (reps) to 8 to 14 per set. At week 3 start progressively increasing your resistance and exercise type.

3. Try hard iron weights if you get tired of the elastic bands.

4. When you get bored with hard iron, try the machines if they are available.

5. You begin to see that there is really no reason to allow yourself to stop.

Important point, if you cannot keep the proper body form doing the resistance for 8 reps, the resistance is probably too heavy.

Remember to change the list of exercises each week or every other week. The change in exercise routines force your muscles to adapt to many different demands and in the end provide more protection to your body.

CORE SERIES OF EXERCISES

The following section will show you a series of exercises Patty and I refer to as a "CORE SERIES OF EXERCISES", for you to use as you begin your training and to return to whenever you wish to "tune-up" your body. These exercises form the foundation for fitness, which in our case we have chosen to target strengthening and stabilizing those core areas of our bodies that give us the greatest support.

In the exercises that follow we show examples we both use that strengthen the muscles and joints of the pelvis, knees, and shoulder girdle. We recommend you become familiar with these exercises, then find other sources for extending a fitness program as you desire.

Common natural weak areas for many people, old or young, are the low back, neck, knees; joints such as elbows, wrists and ankles are other weak points. The CORE SERIES OF EXERCISES will work your muscles to build structural integrity in those potential weak areas. We selected these examples for the above reasons. The volume, duration and intensity are shown at the end of the photo/explanations and are meant to be adjusted by YOUR OWN LEVEL OF ABILITY!

As we have mentioned in other areas, always start with a MINIMUN OF A 10 MINUTE WARM-UP!

Remember to warm-up using the SUN SALUTATION. You can easily make the SUN SALUTATION into a 10 minute routine by repeating the sequence of positions. You may also want to add favorites of your own to increase the warm-up to 10 minutes.

Following the SUN SALUTATION, Patty uses a tread-mill at the Navy Base. I ride my bicycle, run a short distance or perform specific warm-up exercises on the CONCEPT2 ® Indoor Rower. Rowing the ERG (Indoor Rower) is the first choice warm-up for both of us.

Following the warm up we recommend you perform a simple, no load – body weight only, squat keeping your back as straight as possible. We use this squat exercise because it so closely resembles the daily function of sitting and standing. Look around you in church, at movies, in parking lots, in malls, you will see many people struggling to stand up!!! Many of these

Strength

people are in their 40s, 50s and 60s...way too young to be crippled due to non-use of their muscles and joints.

Performing the Body Weight Squat properly will develop spinal and pelvic stability and strength. Add a Standing Leg Press with the rubber bands to add more strength to your legs. Remember to focus as much as possible on keeping your abdominal and oblique muscle core as stable as possible.

Follow along with the remaining strengthening exercises as shown in the photos, keeping in mind stabilizing the body core at all times. End your routine with 10 minute cardiovascular work and record what you did during this session. Perform some light AGE DEFYING stretching from the BICYCLING OR ROWING sections of this book and remember to drink at least 8 ounces of water...and you have started on a life-time of AGE DEFYING STRENGTH TRAINING!

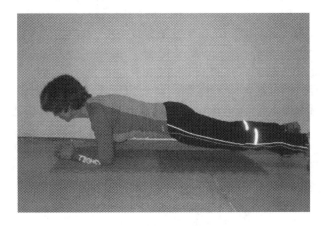

Horizontal Plank hold for 30-60 sec.

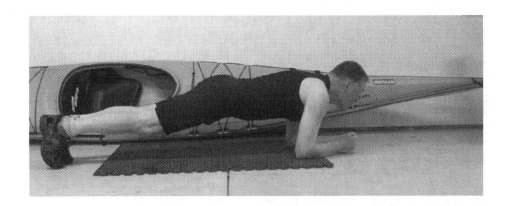

The rubber bands used in the following exercises are the two examples show below.

The examples are SPRI brand exercise bands, however, there are many other brands of exercise bands that work just as well.

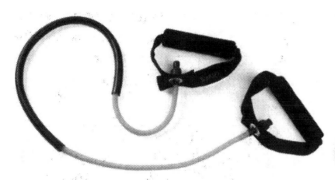

This band is the long band you see me using in the photos. These bands are about 5 feet long and come in the standard strength resistances

The band below has many names depending on the manufacturer. This band by SPRI is known as the Ultra Toner. I have carried these types of bands with me for the past 30 years. The other name for these is the figure eight band. These also come in the standard strength resistances.

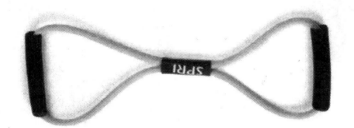

http://www.ehow.com/way_5608276_elastic-band-shoulder-exercises.html

The above web site is an EHOW web site that will instruct you about how to use the rubber band type resistance equipment. There are many other web sites that will give good instruction.

We suggest you spend some time to determine what your specific goals will be.

The examples that follow are just one series that Patty and I have used to target specific muscle areas we tend to use. Some of these exercises target muscles we use less frequently and are therefore helped to keep strong using the rubber band exercises.

CHEST PRESS

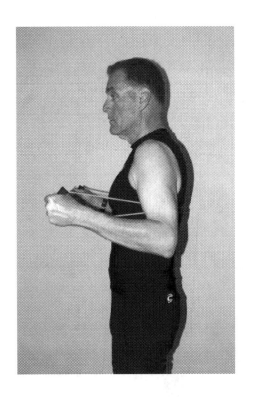 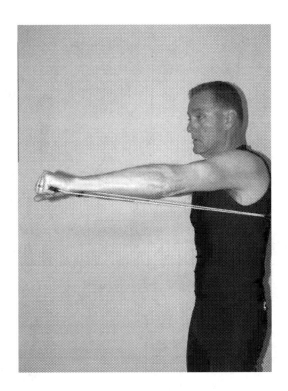

Stand with feet,hip width apart, knees slightly bent. Grasp the handles and place the rubber band behind your back below the shoulder blades. Position your hands just outside your shoulder width palms facing in as shown.

Press arms forward, rotating shoulders ending with palms facing down. Return to start and repeat.

BICEPS CURL

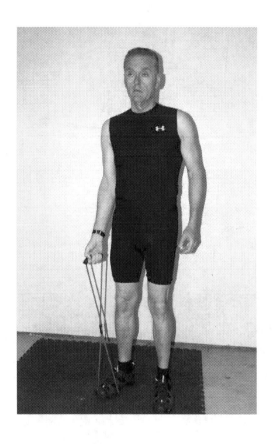 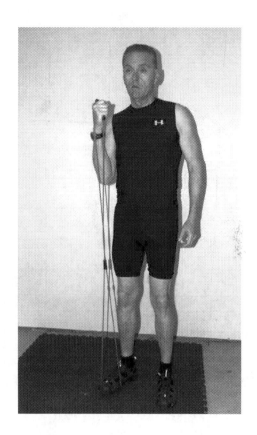

Stand in a staggered stance with rubber band secured under front foot. Grasp the opposite handle with one hand and straighten arm along side of body.

Bend elbow and lift lower arm up and toward chest, keep your elbow close in toward your side. Control the rubber band back to the start position. Keep your back straight, do not sway and do not swing back and forth as you raise the hand against the resistance. If it is too difficult select a less resistive band.

STANDING CHEST ADDUCTION

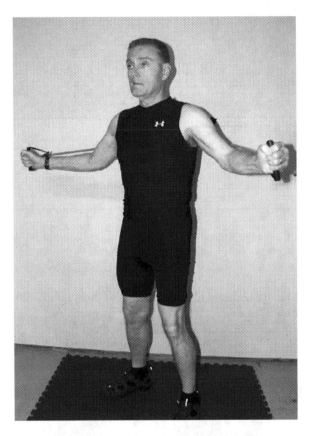 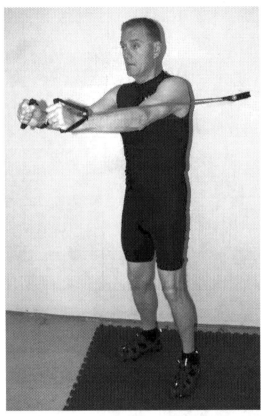

Stand with legs equal distance apart stance. Tighten your core muscles to resist the rubber band. Standing Chest Adduction targets the muscles in the chest, especially the sternal pectorialis major with minor benefit to the anterior deltoids.

In this series of photos I have attached the "door strap" for my SPRI bands to a wall with a sheet rock screw and washer. Normally I would close the "door strap" in a door and thread the tubing through the holder. It works the same either way...probably not good to drill holes in hotel walls...???!!!

Bring your arms up and out to each side. Then bring the arms together in the center of your body. Do not sway or rock your body.

Control the movement out from the sides and return.

Again remember to stabilize the body with your core muscles and legs.

Triceps Extension

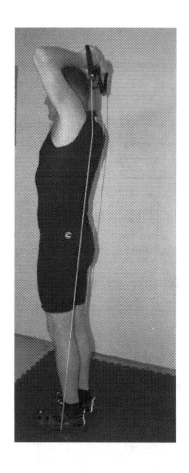 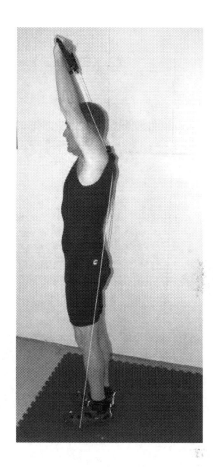

Stand with feet stabilized shoulder width apart. Anchor the rubber band with both feet. Begin with handles behind the head with tension on the rubber bands to keep them aligned between the shoulder blades.

Tighten up your core muscles to keep control of the rubber bands. Extend your arms directly above your head. Control the movement with the triceps muscles.

Control the return of the handles to behind your head. Keep your core straight and controlled. Do not sway or bend at the waist.

Shoulder Press

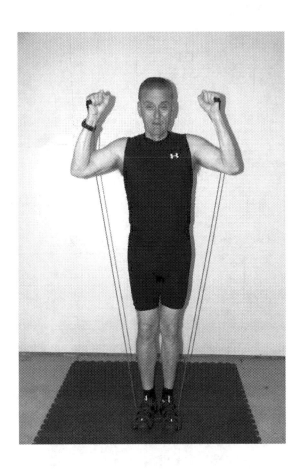 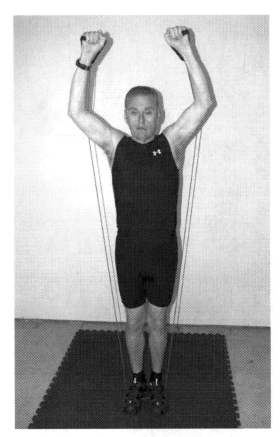

Stand on the rubber band with feet shoulder width apart. As with all rubber band exercises, tighten your abdominal muscles. Grasp each handle as shown with palms facing outward, hands approximately above your elbows, handles about the height of your ears.

Slowly begin pressing your arms above your head. DO NOT lock your knees. Remember to breathe. STOP the upward motion before your elbows are completely straight.
Slowly, in a controlled manner, lower your hands until you return to the start position.

Upright Row

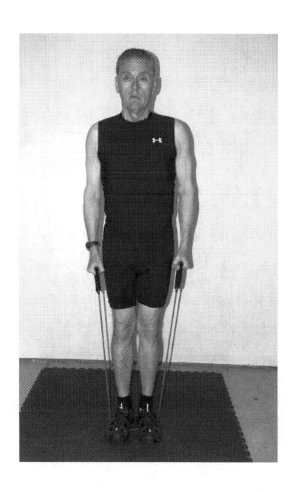 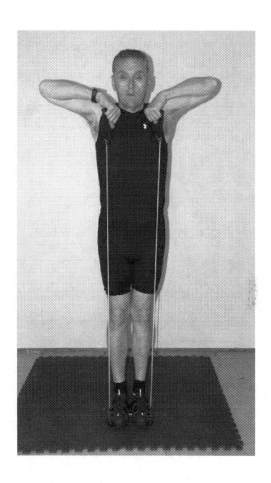

Stand with feet together, mild tension on the rubber band, abdominal muscles tightened. With a slow and controlled movement bring the hands up the front sides of the body with your hands moving in a straight line, moving towards your chin. Try to keep equal pressure and distance between your hands. Do not swing forward to shrug the shoulders while raising the hands. Note how my wrists are controlling the rubber band and the lifting process.

Keep the elbows extended and high. Once you reach as high as you are comfortable going...without going higher than your chin...control the return of the rubber band to the starting position.

This exercise targets a number of muscles

Lateral Rises

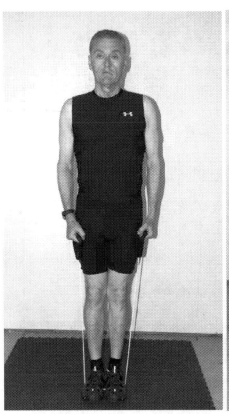 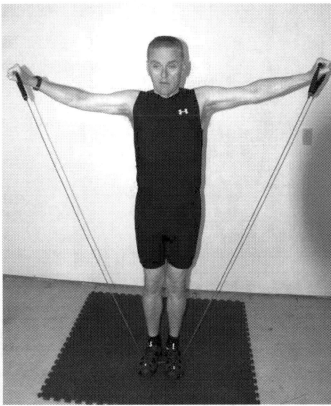

Lateral rises use many of the muscles in the chest, shoulder and deltoid area. The movement is an abduction and adduction movement. Involved in the movement are the trapezius, infraspinatus, latissimus dorsi and pectoralis as well as other minor muscles.

The movement will build the shoulder muscle strength and add stability to the upper body.

Start with arms at sides with mid tension on the rubber bands. Keep arms straight as you raise arms upward. Control arms going up. Do not swing your body backward or forward.

Raise arms slowly until they are parallel to the floor. Lower arms in a smooth controlled manner.

Seated Lat Row

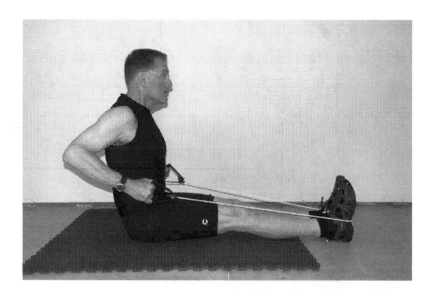

Seated Lat Row is a multi-joint exercise that targets the middle and upper back. Muscles involved are, latissimus dorsi , midtrapezius, and rhomboids.

The entire spine is targeted in this exercise and is therefore an excellent exercise for good posture. This exercise is an excellent base program exercise to assist the core muscles in keeping an individual in good posture position.

Insure rubber band is secure in arch of foot. Keep seated erect, reach out with arms straight, contract core muscles, pull hands into midsection. Do not rotate shoulders down. Pull back with muscles not body swing.

Standing Reverse Back Flyes

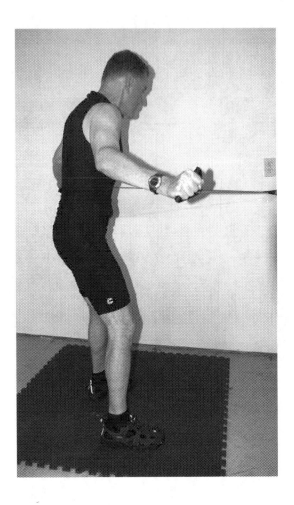

Standing reverse back flyes are an exercise targeting the rear deltoids and the mid-trapezius muscles.

The action of stabilizing your body against the rubber band tension will work your lower body muscles and help with balance control.

Stand with rubber band anchored to spot directly in front of you and about shoulder height. Make a stable stance, contract core muscles for stability, keep arms straight and move hands away from medial point of body toward each side of body.

Hold briefly and return in a controlled manner to the start position. Through entire movement use core muscles to stabilize the body and help resist body movement.

Rubber Band Resisted Squats

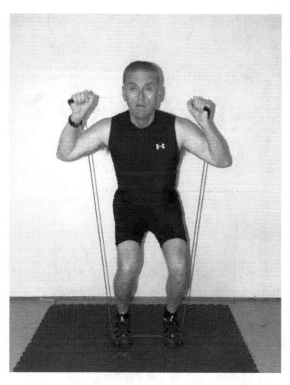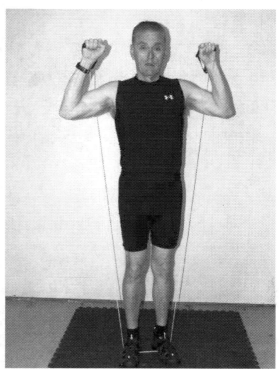

Squats are an exercise that targets the upper leg muscles and the hips. Muscles targeted are the Gluteus, Hamstrings and Quadriceps groups. Also targeted are a series of minor muscles in the hips and legs that allow us all to walk, stand-up, balance on a surf board or play with our grand-children.

The rubber band action in this squat puts no extra weight on the person's shoulders. Almost all of the resistance goes directly into the targeted muscles from the rubber bands

Please remember that in this exercise as well as many other leg exercises, a 90 degree angle between upper and lower leg is the preferred angle. In other words it is not necessary to squat so low that you can touch your heels with your buttocks.

There is no scientific proof that a greater than 90 degree angle will benefit the exerciser. Keep the resistance weight over the ankles, knees aligned with the feet, shoulders back.

Work up to 1 Set of 10 reps with desired resistance.

PLANKS

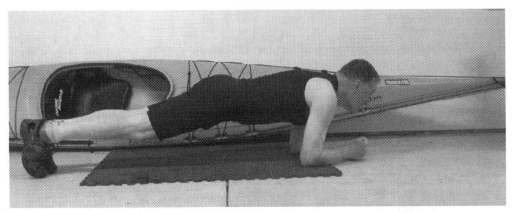

FLAT

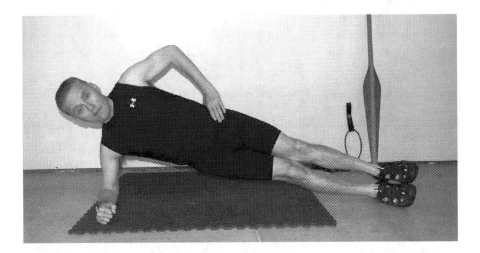

SIDE

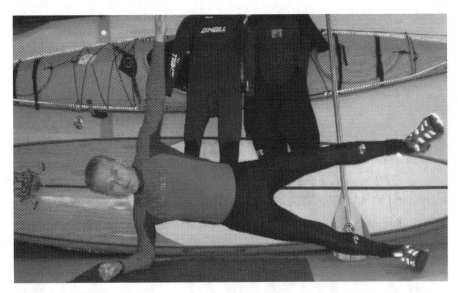

SIDE with LEG LIFT
Jere age 62 with Stand-Up- Paddle Surf Board, wet suit & paddle

THE PLANK

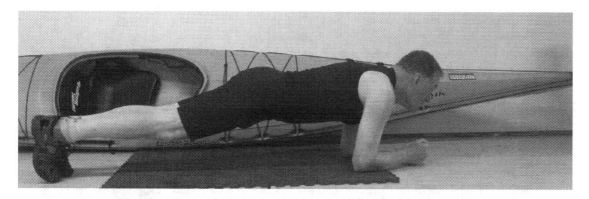

The Plank is a multiple muscle builder aimed at strengthening the "core" muscles as well as the shoulder and back muscles, with legs muscles providing stabilization for the position. This exercise should be an almost everyday exercise.

For 99% of the population the muscles in the body core are challenged as stabilizers for all muscles involved in the activities of Bicycling and Rowing. Each of the sports depends greatly on the strength of the core as developed in The Plank and Side Plank resistance exercise. The Plank, the Humbler Side-Plank and Side Plank With Leg Rise are important to learn and use! Without strong core muscles Bicycling, Rowing and All Activities of Daily Living (ADLs) would be almost impossible.

Begin the exercise with body resting on elbows with elbows under your shoulders. The weight of lower body is supported on toes. Begin to raise your body off the knees by contracting your abdominal muscles, rectus abdominal muscles and the erector spinae muscles. Once off the floor keep your body in a straight line with your head, shoulders, buttocks and feet. You will feel the following muscles engage during the plank, gluteus maximus, deltoids, trapezius, internal obliques, psoas and external obliques.

Start slowly with this exercise. **YOU MUST REMEMBER TO BREATHE!!** Do not hold your breath during this exercise because you can cause a dangerous spike in heart rate, or pass out from lack of oxygen!

Try to stay off the floor in correct position for even 10 seconds when you start. Do not raise your buttocks high in the air...do not allow your back to droop down to the floor. Both of these errors can injure your back. Work up the strength to be able to hold the plank for 15 to 45 seconds. Ultimately you should be able to hold the plank easily for one minute.

SIDE PLANK (THE "HUMBLER")

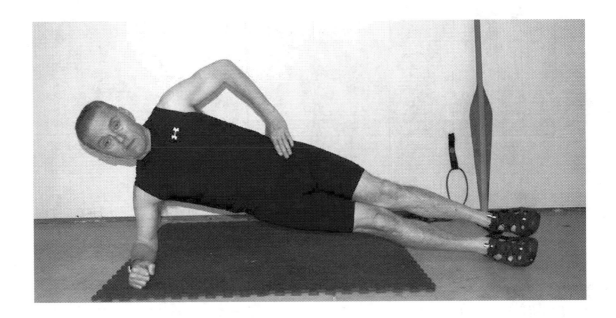

The static exercise known as the Humbler Side Plank strengthens the CORE MUSCLES including the psoas abdominal, back and shoulders. Isometric strength stabilizes the body core.

The abdominal plank is excellent for strengthening transverses abdominal muscles. Transverse abdominal muscles are some of the deepest abdominal muscle layers that include the psoas, and wrap around the entire midsection.

When you contract the abdominals your waist becomes naturally thinner.

(Why isn't EVERY 60 year old doing this exercise every day?)

Therefore, a strong transverse abdominus means a smaller, tighter waist.

Just remember to contract your abdominals in a straight line AND REMEMBER TO BREATHE! You will soon see why this exercise is named "The Humbler".

Start slow, work up to holding the position for 15 – 45 seconds.

Side Plank With Leg Rise

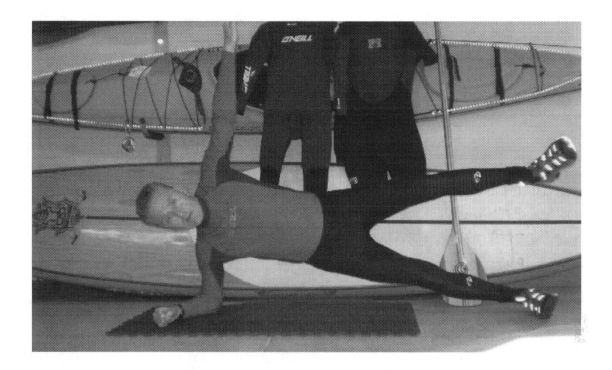

Jere performing the Side Plank with Leg Rise held for 15 to 30 seconds.

The psoas is one of the biggest muscles in your body. It's attached to the vertebrae of your lower back, as well as to your femur. The psoas is mainly involved in hip and thigh movements and can be the source of problems for many people, particularly those who sit for prolonged periods of time.

The side plank is a great exercise that works your core, hip and thigh muscles. The side plank can help you build the psoas muscle, as well as your core stabilizer muscles in your mid-section region. To perform a side plank, lie on the ground on your side. Lift your legs up and keep your body straight as you rest your weight on your forearm. Hold the position for 15 – 30 seconds (or more if you're in good shape). Switch sides and repeat.

Balance

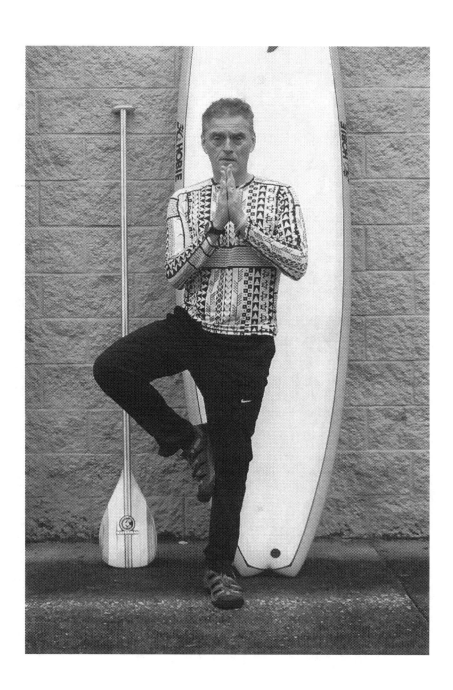

Balance

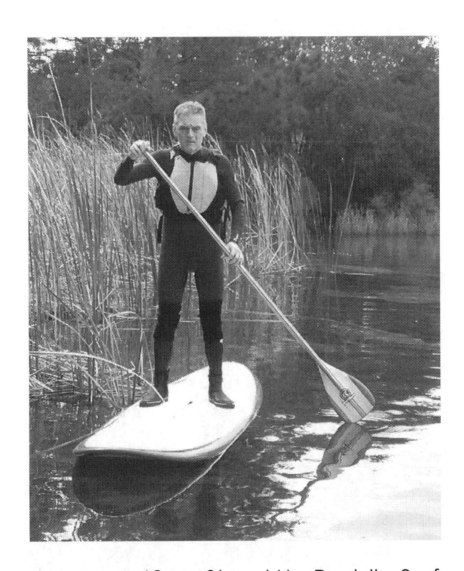

Jere age 62 on Stand Up Paddle Surf Board paddling out to ocean from Jacksonville Beach, Florida.

As with all exercises in this book, consult with your health care provider before attempting ANY of these balance training exercises.

Patty and I train with balance exercises each day. We often use our home gym or the Navy Base Gym at N. A. S. Jacksonville. The following photos and exercises are a small part of our daily and weekly balance training.

These are what Patty and I call balance poses. Perhaps they are also yoga poses; however, we refer to these as balance poses. Remember, your body balances itself using many small muscles to keep you in a static upright position. Once you start to practice true balance while standing straight up you will sense many small muscles in your body contracting and loosening while they attempt to keep you upright. Most of these contractions are almost automatic.

Start out slowly following the photos, even if you can only get part way into the pose you are advancing. Only go as far into the pose as you feel safe. Perform your practice with a chair, sofa, table or other stable object you can hold on to while you start your balance training.

One leg prayer balance:

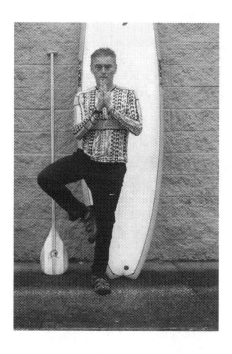

Balance

I have been using the two balance positions below for almost 40 years. I learned these while I was in Graduate School of Architecture at the University of Illinois in Champaign, Il. One of the Grad Student's mother was a YOGA teacher. She often visited him and would teach us ways to relax from the constant strain of mathematics, design and art studies. For some reason this particular pose stuck in my brain and I use it today just about every day.

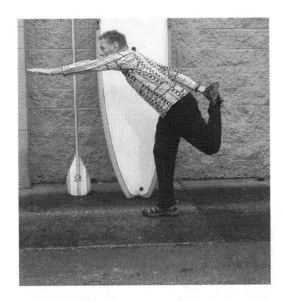

Balance left leg, stretch right leg.

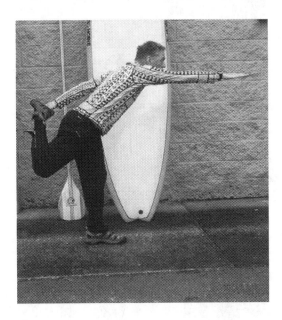

Balance on right leg, stretch left leg.

Work up slowly to be able to hold these positions for 15, 30, 45 and 60 seconds.

As we get older our ability to be aware of our balance becomes even more important. American College of Sports Medicine reports the current yearly hospital admission for broken hips is around 300,000.

On the day that our grand-daughter, Alice, was born, I started back surfing. I chose to return to surfing using a Stand-Up-Paddle (SUP)surf board.

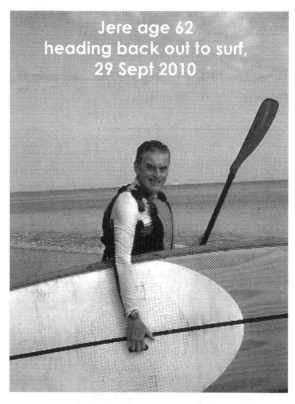

Jere age 62 heading back out to surf, 29 Sept 2010

So, on 7 May 2010, at 0700 in the morning I set out upon the ocean off Jacksonville, Beach, Florida and returned to surfing.

Just one hour later Alice was born and I met Alice about 5 hours later.

The balance required to surf on a Stand Up Paddle board is extremely good balance training. I had practiced on flat water lakes before trying the ocean surf. When I did get into the ocean it was great!

The idea of being able to SUP at age 62 may seem just a little extreme. However, since I have begun I have met several male and female SUP ocean surfers who are 10 and 15 years older than I am!!!! That means these people are 72 and 77 years old!

We can all agree that Endurance and Strength training are vital to keeping aging baby-boomers healthy and active. Now we can add that balance training is equally important.

A very good source for balance training information is the excellent book by Dr. Steven P. Weiniger, STAND TALLER – LIVE LONGER...AN ANTI-AGING STRATEGY.

In addition to SUP surfing in the ocean, when the weather gets stormy or cold I use a BOSU ® Ball in our home gym or the gym at the Navy Base. This BOSU ball is an excellent balance trainer. www.bosu.com There are many other books and training devices available that are just as good as these mentioned.

Balance

The important issue is to continue training your muscles and overall body to remember how to balance!

BOSU Ball balance: Look at these following photos and decide if you want to try them on flat ground first. Once you feel comfortable on flat ground NOT on the BOSU try the balancing on the BOSU. Start on the BOSU where you are near an object you can use to help balance if you feel you may fall.

As you balance on the BOSU feel the many small muscles within your body working to keep you upright. These are the muscles you want to train. Once you feel confident work on the deep knee bends, Your back, hips, groin and thigh muscle will feel great and you will be on your way to a new life of pain free walking.

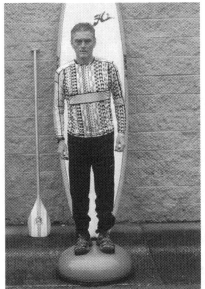

1. Find a good balance stance.

One of the people in the Navy gym is 88 years old. He uses the BOSU ball every time I see him in the gym. He is amazing!

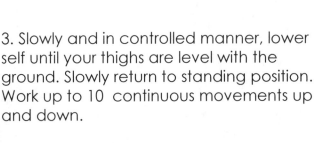

2. Extend arms for balance.

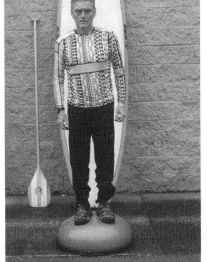

3. Slowly and in controlled manner, lower self until your thighs are level with the ground. Slowly return to standing position. Work up to 10 continuous movements up and down.

BOSU Ball balance: Look at these following photos and decide if you want to try them on flat ground first. These balance exercises on the BOSU are done while balancing an object on the extended finger tips. In these photos I am balancing my Stand Up Paddle Board paddle across my finger tips as I move from standing position to full crouch with thighs level with ground.

Go slowly. Keep your eyes looking STRAIGHT AHEAD!!!!!

NEVER LOOK DOWN at the ground or the BOSU ball...you will lose your balance.

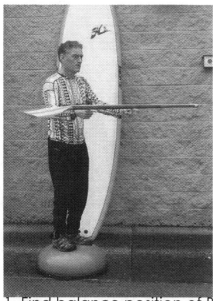

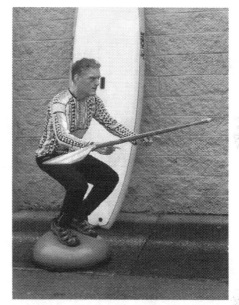

1. Find balance position of BOSU ball. Balance oar or other straight pole object on finger tips. DO NOT LOOK DOWN...YOU WILL FALL!!!!

2. Ease yourself down keeping the oar balanced on your finger tips arms straight out in front.

3. Once you are down in the crouch position, hold the position and feel your muscles as they work to balance your body.

Initially your legs will tremble. However, with time and training you will be able to accomplish this move and feel very good about your improved ability to balance!

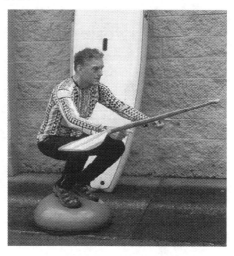

Tracking

◊   How Much Exercise Should I Get?

◊   Weekly Schedule

◊   Balance & Strength Chart

◊   Daily Record

How much exercise should I get each week?

When you first start out, you might have trouble keeping up with even the minimum amount of exercise we suggest in the chart at the bottom. Start out with a schedule that your body can tolerate and that you think you really can manage and build up from there. Note that the schedules are arranged so that you are never doing strength exercises of the same muscle groups on any two days in a row. If you want to do strength exercises every day, alternate muscle groups. For example, do strength exercises of your upper-body muscles on Monday, Wednesday and Friday and of your lower-body muscles on Tuesday, Thursday and Saturday. Or you can do strength exercises of all of your muscle groups up to every other day. Begin exercising gradually.

Once you have worked you way up to a regular schedule....

...get at least this much exercise each week:

Sunday	Monday	Tuesday	Wednesday	Thursday	Friday	Saturday
Stretching	Endurance	Strength/ balance, all muscle groups	Endurance Stretching	Strength/ balance, all muscle groups	Endurance	Stretching

Weekly Schedule

You may want to make copies of this form. Leave this one blank, so you can copy it as needed. Write in the exercises and activities you plan to do. Create a schedule you think you really can manage. You can change your plan as your fitness improves and you are able to do more.

Week of:	Endurance	Strength	Flexibility	Balance
Sunday				
Monday				
Tuesday				
Wednesday				
Thursday				
Friday				
Saturday				

Balance and Strength

BALANCE AND STRENGTH. You may want to make copies of this form. Leave this one blank, so you can copy it as needed. This form is for keeping track of the activities and exercises you do each day.

Week of	Sunday	Monday	Tuesday	Wednesday	Thursday	Friday	Saturday
Endurance: List the activity you did and how long you did it.							
Flexibility: Check the box of each stretching exercise you did:							

Daily Record

ANYTIME, ANYWHERE BALANCE. You may want to make copies of this form. Leave this one blank, so you can copy it as needed. This form is for keeping track of the activities and exercises you do each day.

Week of	Sunday	Monday	Tuesday	Wednesday	Thursday	Friday	Saturday
Anytime, anywhere balance. Check the box of each exercise you did:							
Stand on one foot Left Right							
Stand and sit without using hands							
Walk heel - to - toe							

Muscles Diagram

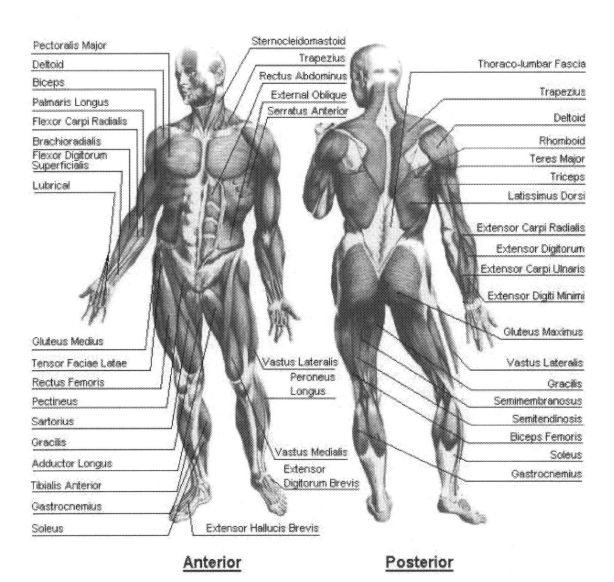

Pectoralis Major
Deltoid
Biceps
Palmaris Longus
Flexor Carpi Radialis
Brachioradialis
Flexor Digitorum Superficialis
Lubrical

Sternocleidomastoid
Trapezius
Rectus Abdominus
External Oblique
Serratus Anterior

Thoraco-lumbar Fascia
Trapezius
Deltoid
Rhomboid
Teres Major
Triceps
Latissimus Dorsi

Gluteus Medius
Tensor Faciae Latae
Rectus Femoris
Pectineus
Sartorius
Gracilis
Adductor Longus
Tibialis Anterior
Gastrocnemius
Soleus

Vastus Lateralis
Peroneus Longus

Vastus Medialis
Extensor Digitorum Brevis

Extensor Hallucis Brevis

Extensor Carpi Radialis
Extensor Digitorum
Extensor Carpi Ulnaris
Extensor Digiti Minimi
Gluteus Maximus
Vastus Lateralis
Gracilis
Semimembranosus
Semitendinosis
Biceps Femoris
Soleus
Gastrocnemius

Anterior   **Posterior**

122

Notes:

Resources APPENDIX

Books:

Carmichael, Chris & Edmund Burke. Fitness Cycling. Human Kinetics Publishers Inc. 1994

National Institute of Aging Publication: fitness over fifty. Hatherleigh Press. 2003

Dr. Steven P. Weiniger. STAND TALL~LIVE LONGER. Published by BodyZone LLC. 2008

Internet WEB Sites:

Concept2 Rowing: www.concept.com

BOSU Ball: www.BOSU.com

SPRI : www.spri.com

Courses :

Master Fitness Specialist: Cooper Institute Aerobic Research (CIAR), Dallas, Texas, 2003.

Health Promotion Director: Cooper Institute Aerobic Research (CIAR), Dallas, Texas, 1998.

Master's Degree; Master of Sciences; Community Health and Wellness (CHW): California College of Health Science, Los Angeles, CA; 2000. (Graduated with Honors)

American College of Sports Medicine: Bi-Monthly Continuing Education Credits (CEC's) 1990 to present